I0705273

Contents

Preface

Who's this book for?

As societal trends increasingly emphasize physical appearance, retinoids like Isotretinoin (brand name Accutane) have become a popular solution for acne and fine wrinkles. However, as the use of these medications becomes more widespread, so does awareness of their potential side effects. For most people without a medical background, their understanding of retinoids and Vitamin A is often limited to knowing they are found in red and orange foods like carrots and play a role in vision. Yet, for those unfortunate enough to experience complications, they soon realize that Vitamin A affects nearly all biological processes. The side effects of retinoid medications can impact muscles and joints, vision, the digestive system, and, most concerning, the brain. This book focuses on that final, and perhaps most alarming, category of side effects.

Some mental health disturbances caused by retinoids may be relatively mild, such as increased fatigue or agitation. However, there have been instances of much more severe reactions, particularly with isotretinoin, including psychosis. One of the more perplexing, and still unexplained, side effects is a lasting loss of sexual desire, which may be linked to a broader sense of apathy.

Understanding how retinoids can cause cognitive disturbances, or any of their peripheral effects, is no easy task—especially since the science behind these phenomena is still emerging. Patients seeking answers from their healthcare providers often receive unsatisfactory explanations, which can lead to even greater frustration and despair. That's where this book aims to help. While it's impossible to explain the broad and sometimes severe side effects of retinoid medications without understanding the underlying science, I've provided a layman-friendly approach that makes this material accessible, even to readers with only a basic grasp of biology. One way I've achieved this is by summarising the key points of each subchapter into concise bullet points, offering a clear takeaway.

Each chapter of this book explores how retinoids function within the body and outlines the known effects of retinoid medications. However, as previously mentioned, understanding precisely how a drug like isotretinoin can produce such dramatic impacts on mental health remains beyond current scientific knowledge. Over the past few decades, researchers have attempted to solve this mystery, with studies indicating changes in brain activity within the prefrontal cortex and alterations in serotonin receptor expression. I have presented this research while also providing the foundational knowledge needed to understand it. Additionally, I offer my own hypotheses on the neurological effects of retinoids, based on research into the retinoic acid pathway, which has yet to be directly linked to the adverse effects of retinoid medications. These hypotheses are supported by hundreds of studies.

Retinoids appear to influence neurological health in many ways, affecting dopamine, serotonin, neuronal growth, and more, making it difficult to pinpoint which mechanism primarily explains isotretinoin's impact on the brain. It's possible that one specific effect may be more relevant for some individuals than others, but it's impossible to know for certain. That's why I've explored all potential pathways individually, while acknowledging that only one may ultimately explain the mood-related side effects of isotretinoin. For each category I examine, I also highlight medications and supplements known to have inverse effects on those systems. In some cases, this understanding may offer insights into how adverse effects might be prevented or reversed.

This book should not be seen as the definitive answer to how isotretinoin can profoundly alter mental health in certain patients, as it reflects only our current scientific understanding, and new discoveries may emerge in the future. Nevertheless, I am confident that this book provides the most comprehensive exploration of the topic, drawing on hundreds of individual studies and analyses. For those suffering from potentially long-lasting side effects of medications like isotretinoin, I hope this book offers both valuable insights and reassurance.

1. Introduction

1.1 A Billion Dollar Industry

Retinoids are increasingly becoming a staple for many people's cosmetic routines, with different formulations offering permanent relief acne to reducing the appearance of skin aging. Retinoids are either natural or synthetic chemicals that are structurally related to vitamin A and are available in both over the counter formulations such as retinol creams, or as prescription medications such as Isotretinoin. Over the next ten years the global retinoid market is projected to almost double, from $1.63 billion to $3 billion. [4] The cosmetic benefits of retinoid treatment are enticing, in particular reducing the appearance of skin aging.

All cells in the body (aside from sperm and ova) have an in-built life span, predetermining the number of times it can divide, and repair based on telomere length. Telomeres are essentially protective end caps at the end of chromosomes which ensure that when DNA is replicated, the important genetic information is not lost. When cells divide the telomeres shorten slightly, and over time the telomeres become critically short at which point the cell enters senescence and can no longer divide – a point called the Hayflick limit. This is the reality of aging, and at least as it is currently understood it cannot be avoided. After dividing between 50-100 times, keratinocytes (the principal cells in the skin) reach this point of cellular senescence. [5]

Whilst there's little disagreement that retinoids do offer relief from the appearance of skin aging, there's still some debate as to how they achieve this. In both long- and short-term studies, topical retinoids reduce the appearance of photoaging at a variety of doses. [6] This includes improvements in skin texture, hyperpigmentation and fine wrinkling. One of the proposed mechanisms is that retinoids improve collagen formation by blocking the effect of collagenase, which is the enzyme that breaks down collagen. [7] Additionally, retinoids profoundly alter the pattern of differentiation and proliferation not only of skin cells, but in tissues throughout the body – which will be explored at length throughout this book.

Cell proliferation and differentiation are interconnected processes through which stem-like cells contribute to tissue growth and specialization. Stem cells can proliferate to produce more stem cells, aiding in growth and replenishment, or they can differentiate into specialized tissue cells with a more limited capacity for replication. Proliferation is essential for increasing cell numbers and maintaining cell populations, while differentiation transforms these cells into specialized types with specific functions—such as skin or muscle cells. A crucial balance between these two processes must be carefully regulated to ensure proper development, maintenance, and aging of tissues. Retinoids appear to both be able to encourage differentiation and also programmed cell death, called apoptosis, in keratinocytes. [8]

1.2 'Post Accutane Syndrome'

The effects of Retinoids like Accutane are broad and complex, just as the roles of endogenous retinoic acid are widespread throughout the body, influencing skin health, differentiation and proliferation, eye health, the immune system, neurological functions, bone growth and the gut. A full appreciation of all the ways in which Accutane impacts all these systems would not only make this book tediously long but is also fundamentally limited by the current scientific understanding, with the literature on some of these interactions being relatively scarce. For this reason, the primary focus of this book will be on the neurological effects of Accutane, although some of these peripheral effects will also be touched upon.

Whilst many different retinoid formulations are available, the most popular retinoid is Isotretinoin, also known by its brand name Accutane. Over the years, its effectiveness in treating severe acne has been well-documented, earning it a reputation as a potent solution where other treatments fail. However, alongside its efficacy in treating acne, it has also been associated with a range of potential side effects—particularly in relation to the brain. However, just as Accutane can offer permanent relief from acne, so too can the side effects appear to be permanent for some unlucky patients.

The extent of its psychological impact gained prominence during a 2015 murder trial, where attorneys argued that a 15-year-old experienced homicidal psychosis as a result of his treatment with the acne drug. [1] Though this may seem far-fetched, it isn't an isolated incident, and the connection between Vitamin A and neurological disorders has long been recognized.

The effects of overexposure to Vitamin A on the central nervous system were first documented in 1856 by Elisha Kane, an Arctic explorer who suffered dramatic changes in mood and temperament after ingesting polar bear liver. Many symptoms of Accutane treatment significantly overlap with those of Hypervitaminosis A, as Accutane exerts its therapeutic effects through the primary metabolite of Vitamin A: Retinoic Acid. However, unlike overexposure to Vitamin A, isotretinoin avoids xenobiotic responses that metabolize excessive retinoic acid, allowing for even greater intracellular accumulation. [2]

A meta-analysis of 25 randomized controlled trials found that neurological symptoms were among the most common adverse effects associated with Accutane treatment, with 24% of patients suffering from extreme fatigue and 10% reporting significant changes in mood and personality. [3] The most disturbing and enigmatic of these neurological effects is the apparent impact on sexual functioning, often termed 'Post-Retinoid Sexual Dysfunction'

(PRSD). This disturbing ramification of treatment with Retinoid medications has even prompted the European Medicines Agency to recommend that erectile dysfunction be added to the product information of Isotretinoin products in 2017. [9]

There have been proposed diagnostic criteria for this specific reaction based on reports of complete loss of interest in sexual activities, as well as diminished genital sensitivity. [10] The overlap of these symptoms with those resulting from the popular hair loss medication Finasteride has also highlighted the possible significance of changes to endocrine function, with both testosterone and it's more potent metabolite DHT (Dihydrotestosterone) also being impacted by the acne drug.

Whilst so-called 'Post Accutane Syndrome' is yet to have a formal characterisation by doctors, the collection of anecdotal reports and testimonies paints a picture of enduring anhedonia, including a notable disinterest in sexual behaviour. The reports of psychological changes following treatment with Accutane aren't without strong biological evidence either, with retinoids impacting numerous multiple signalling pathways in the brain, including dopamine, serotonin, GABA and neurogenesis. The evidence and mechanisms involved in each of these pathways will be explored in subsequent chapters.

2. What is Accutane?

To understand the effects of not only Accutane but all Retinoids and Vitamin A itself, you need to fundamentally understand one process: differentiation. To those unfamiliar with biology, this word might provoke trepidation from its use in calculus. However, in the biological context differentiation is fairly self-explanatory. It refers to the process by which stem cells or progenitor cells become distinct and specialised to a particular type of tissue cell. This is the fundamental purpose of Retinoids in the body, to guide the process of differentiation. In this chapter I'll first explain what is meant by the classification of Retinoids, what their function is in the body before explaining what's unique about Accutane.

2.1 What are Retinoids?

Retinoids are the class of chemicals related to vitamin A. They play a role in regulating a wide range of biological systems, including vision, cell proliferation/differentiation, bone tissue, and the immune system. "Retinoid" is a general term that encompasses a range of molecules, including retinol, retinoic acid, and retinyl esters, as well as synthetic retinoids. The breadth of retinoids' effects in the body is perhaps greater than that of any other vitamin. Despite retinoids existing in many forms, most retinoid signalling comes from the primary metabolite all-trans retinoic acid (ATRA). ATRA binds to several types of nuclear receptors, including Retinoic Acid Receptor (RAR), Retinoid X Receptor (RXR), and Peroxisome proliferator-activated receptors (PPARs). [1]

Vitamin A is classified as a dietary vitamin because the body cannot synthesize it on its own. The precursor to vitamin A, beta-carotene, can be obtained from plant sources that possess orange and red colours, such as carrots. Additionally, retinyl esters can be obtained from animal sources, such as beef liver, which is the storage form of vitamin A that accumulates in the liver and adipose fat. [2] These retinyl esters do not have a significant role aside from serving as substrates for conversion into other retinoid products in the body, such as 11-cis-retinal for vision. [3]

Retinol itself does not primarily contribute to the biological roles of vitamin A, as it must first be converted into retinoic acid. [4] It is believed that Accutane also serves as a substrate for conversion into retinoic acid within the cell. The advantage of applying isotretinoin (Accutane) rather than retinoic acid is that it bypasses the body's metabolizing enzymes (P450), which would otherwise break down excessive retinoic acid. This allows for greater accumulation of retinoic acid in the cell nucleus. [5]

While retinol is essential for the healthy functioning of tissues throughout the body, excessive retinol can result in a range of potentially serious conditions. Hypervitaminosis A can damage the same tissues that healthy retinol levels regulate effectively, such as the skin, hair, eyes, brain, and more. Toxic levels of vitamin A are also teratogenic, meaning they cause congenital disabilities in developing foetuses. [6] To prevent the harmful effects of hypervitaminosis A, the body carefully regulates the enzymes that synthesize retinoic acid through a negative feedback mechanism. These enzymes are Aldehyde Dehydrogenases (ALDH) and Retinaldehyde Dehydrogenases (RALDH). [7][8]

2.2 What is Accutane?

Isotretinoin (Accutane) is an isomer of retinoic acid; it occurs naturally in very small doses but primarily exerts its effect through the metabolite all-trans-retinoic acid (ATRA). The advantage of administering isotretinoin rather than simply ATRA is that it has a longer half-life, allowing for less frequent administration. Isotretinoin is distinct from ATRA because it has a cis bond on the 13th carbon.

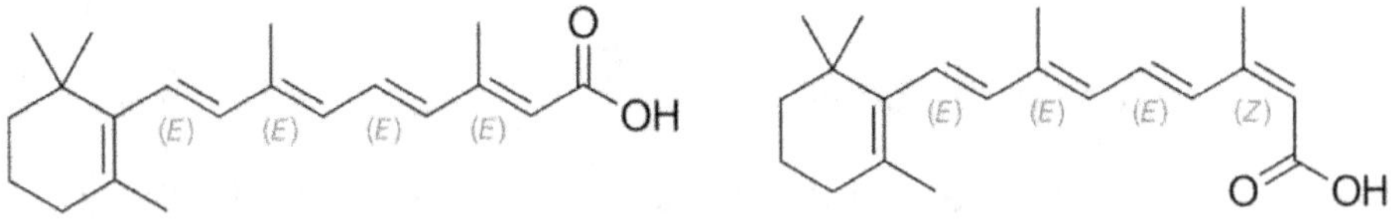

[Fig 1] **All trans retinoic acid (ATRA) vs. cis-13 retinoic acid.** (Vaccinationist, Public domain, via Wikimedia Commons)

The cis-13 form of retinoic acid (13cRA) is not as potent a gene regulator as the more commonly occurring all-trans retinoic acid (ATRA), so Accutane must first undergo full-trans isomerization into ATRA to exert its effects throughout the body. However, taking the Accutane form of retinoic acid may offer some advantages over direct treatment with ATRA. Administering isotretinoin can lead to a higher nuclear concentration (within the cell nucleus) of ATRA than applying ATRA directly. This is because isotretinoin avoids triggering a xenobiotic metabolizing response from cytochrome P450. [13] Once bound to the Retinoic Acid Receptor (RAR), the RXR/RAR heterodimer complex binds to DNA to transcribe retinoic acid response genes. [14]

2.3 Differentiation

Almost every cell in the body undergoes a life cycle that can be broken into four phases. The first stage being G1 (gap 1) phase, which is where the cell synthesises proteins and mRNA to prepare for cell division. Next the S (synthesis phase) takes place, where DNA is replicated to ensure the genome can be perfectly copied across to the new cell. Next follows the G2 (gap 2) phase, where chromatin condenses into chromosomes. The chromatin is the long string of DNA, that first must be packaged into tight structures called chromosomes. Finally, once all this preparation has taken place the cell can divide though mitosis, and a new cell is formed.

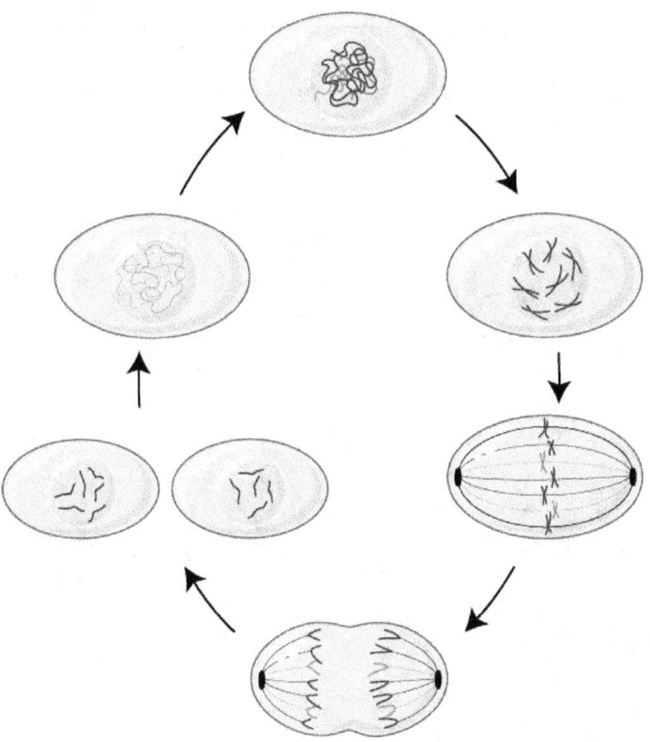

[Fig 2] **Depiction of Mitosis**. (Servier Medical Art is licensed under CC BY 4.0 https://smart.servier.com/smart_image/mitosis/)

The new copy of chromosomes are separated into a new nucleus and new cell is a copy of the first. Cells can be taken outside of this cycle of replication into G0, or quiescent phase. This might occur because there simply isn't sufficient nutrients to support the growth of new cells, or because some cells don't require regeneration unless there is injury. Most cells in adults exist in the G0 phase, and don't need proliferation. For example, cells in the liver very rarely divide, but when a section of liver is surgically removed or damaged, the cells rapidly proliferate to repair the damage.

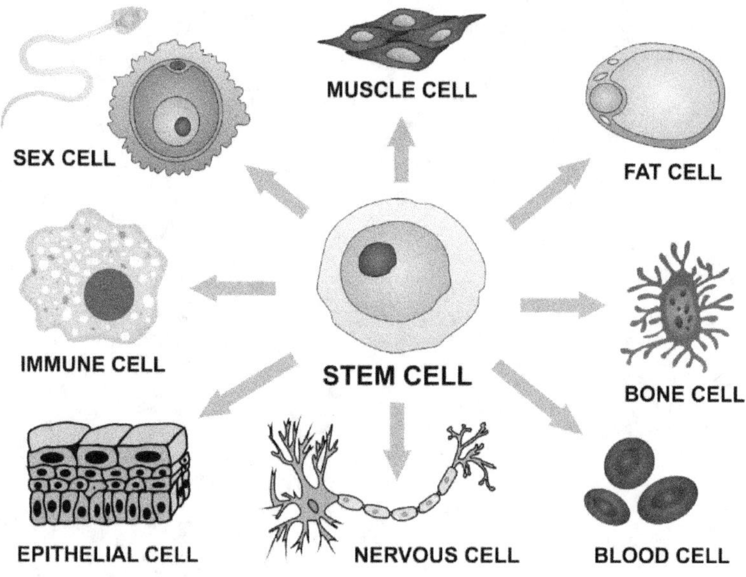

[Fig 3] **Cell Differentiation from stem cells into specialised cells**. (Haileyfournier, CC BY-SA 4.0 <https://creativecommons.org/licenses/by-sa/4.0>, via Wikimedia Commons)

During cell proliferation, tissues growth individual cells grow whilst dividing, and therefor maintain cells of a roughly constant size. If the cells did not also grow as they divide, then the tissue mass would remain constant as it divides into smaller and smaller cells. Cells can also change purpose or function through a process of differentiation. A progenitor or stem cell can become specialised to perform specific tissues or functions. Some cells have a short life span and must be replaced by continual cell proliferation such as blood cells and epithelial cells of the skin or digestive tract.

These cells are not replaced through direct proliferation of the differentiated cells however, instead they proliferate from less differentiated stem cells. Stem cells also divide to produce new stem cells and act as reserve for throughout an entire lifetime. However, some cells can proliferate in an uncontrolled manner and avoid the typical cycle of cell death. These cells are called cancer cells and form tumours that disrupt normal tissue function and can ultimately lead to death.

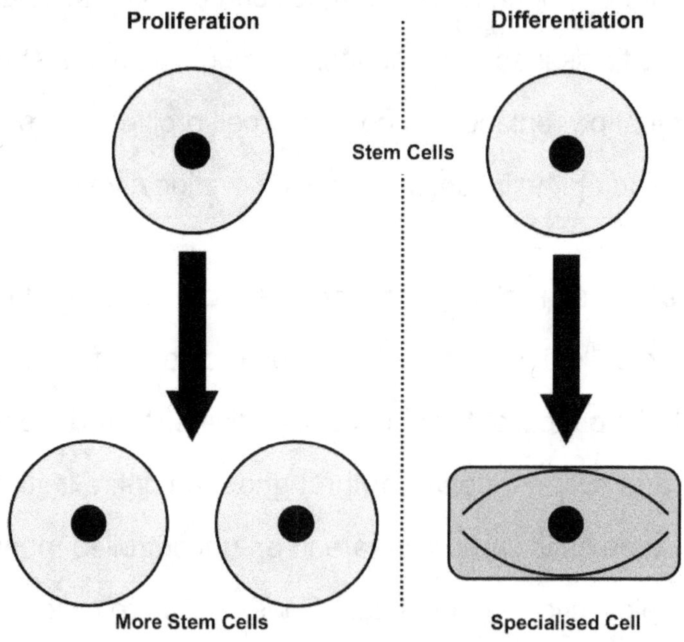

Fig 4] **Cell Proliferation vs. Differentiation**

Where does vitamin A come in? Retinoic acid is needed to help signal for cells to become differentiated and specialised from progenitor or stem cells. However high levels of retinoic acid can directly inhibit cell growth. This is most relevant to foetal development, where cells are rapidly proliferating and differentiating. The mother needs healthy levels of vitamin A ensure that stem cells differentiate appropriately to form new limbs in a process called morphogenesis. The absence of vitamin A leads to uncontrolled proliferation of epithelial stem cells that fail to differentiate. For this reason, there has been a strong interest in retinoids reducing cancer risk.

2.4 How Retinoids Regulate Differentiation

One of the key signalling pathways by which Retinoids influence differentiation is the Wnt/β-catenin pathway. The scope of this growth signalling pathway is broad and is key to understanding the effects of Retinoids more generally through the body. β-catenin is a growth-signalling protein central to the Wnt pathway, which is essential for cell adhesion, tissue growth, development, and homeostasis. β -catenin is a growth-signalling protein central to the Wnt pathway, which plays a key role in cell adhesion, tissue growth, development, and homeostasis. It is essential for maintaining pluripotent stem cell proliferation, and in its absence, these cells undergo differentiation, leading to the loss of their stemness.

Wnt proteins (named 'wingless' due to their shape) activate the 'canonical' Wnt/β-catenin pathway, leading to the transcription of β-catenin target genes. In the absence of Wnt ligands (binding molecules), β-catenin is continuously marked for degradation within a 'destruction complex.'

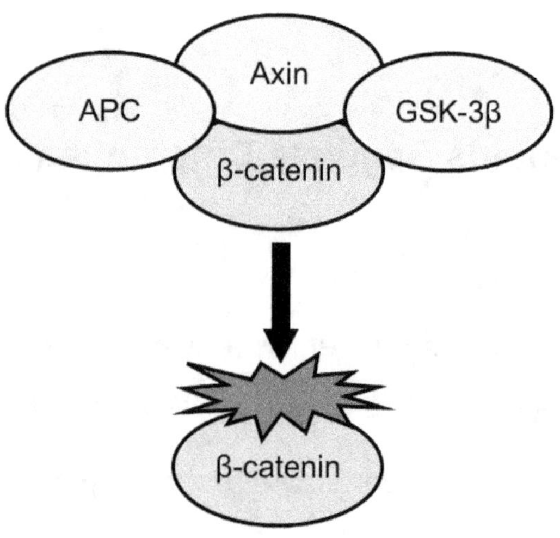

[Fig 5] **The Destruction Complex (Axin, APC, GSK-3β) continuously breaks down β-catenin.**

This destruction complex, which traps β-catenin, consists of Axin, APC, GSK-3β (glycogen synthase kinase 3 beta), and CK1. When Wnt proteins bind to receptors (Frizzled and LRP5/6) on the cell surface, the destruction complex is inhibited, allowing β-catenin to stabilize and accumulate in the cytoplasm. β-catenin then translocates into the nucleus, where it interacts with TCF/LEF transcription factors to regulate the expression of target genes related to cell proliferation and differentiation. [9]

ATRA (the primary active metabolite of Accutane) can block the action of β-catenin by enhancing the destruction complex's activity. ATRA achieves this by inhibiting PI3K-AKT, which upregulates GSK-3β's degradation of β-catenin. [10] Retinoic acid also appears to directly impact the transaction of LEF/TCF by β-catenin, which are the primary transcription factors that mediate the effects of β-catenin. One of β-catenin's key roles is maintaining stem cell populations. When β-catenin activity is blocked, stem cells undergo differentiation, losing their pluripotent self-renewing properties. [11]

One of Accutane's medical applications is in treating cancers, where tumours maintain their self-renewing stem cell properties to rapidly proliferate. ATRA can disrupt tumorigenesis by blocking β-catenin and triggering differentiation. [12] While Accutane exerts this differentiating effect on cancer stem cells, it can also induce differentiation in healthy tissues throughout the body that rely on stem cell populations for maintenance, such as bones, skin, the gut, and the brain.

2.5 Conclusion

In conclusion, Accutane (isotretinoin) exerts a powerful influence over stem cell differentiation and proliferation. By converting into all-trans retinoic acid (ATRA) and bypassing metabolic degradation, Accutane achieves higher nuclear concentrations of ATRA than direct administration of retinoic acid or retinol. This leads to potent modulation of gene transcription through nuclear receptors like RAR and RXR.

Accutane's modulation of stem cell proliferation is particularly owed to its ability to enhance the destruction of β-catenin in the Wnt signalling. This promotes differentiation and inhibits cell proliferation. Whilst this may be beneficial in treating conditions like severe acne and certain cancers by reducing uncontrolled cell growth, it also poses serious risks. The inhibition of β-catenin affects healthy stem cell populations, leading to potential adverse effects on tissues that rely on regular cell renewal, such as the skin, bones, gut, and brain.

Excessive retinoid activity can result in hypervitaminosis A, causing damage to various organs and increasing the risk of teratogenic effects during foetal development. The body's natural regulatory mechanisms are bypassed by Accutane, posing a greater risk than excessive consumption of dietary retinol alone.

2.6 Chapter Summary

- **Essential Roles and Signalling**: Retinoids, related to vitamin A, are crucial for vision, cell growth and differentiation, bone health, and immune function. The primary signalling molecule, all-trans retinoic acid (ATRA), interacts with nuclear receptors such as RAR, RXR, and PPARs to regulate these biological processes.

- **Diverse Forms and Impact:** The retinoid class includes various forms like retinol, retinoic acid, retinyl esters, and synthetic variants. This diversity allows retinoids to have a broader range of effects in the body than any other vitamin.

- **Dietary Sources and Conversion:** Since the body cannot synthesize vitamin A, it must be obtained from the diet. Beta-carotene from colourful plant sources (e.g., carrots) and retinyl esters from animal sources (e.g., beef liver) serve as precursors that are converted into active retinoid compounds necessary for biological functions.

- **Regulation and Toxicity:** Excessive intake of vitamin A can lead to hypervitaminosis A, causing damage to tissues and congenital disabilities. To prevent toxicity, the body regulates retinoic acid synthesis through enzymes like ALDH and RALDH using a negative feedback mechanism.

- **Cell Cycle and Quiescence:** Cells undergo a four-phase life cycle—G1 (protein and mRNA synthesis), S (DNA replication), G2 (chromatin condensation), and mitosis (cell division). Most adult cells enter the G0 phase, a non-dividing state, due to limited need for proliferation unless prompted by factors like injury.

- **Proliferation and Differentiation:** Tissue growth involves cells both growing in size and dividing to maintain constant cell size. Stem and progenitor cells differentiate into specialized cell types to replace short-lived cells, such as blood and skin cells, ensuring tissue maintenance and repair.

- **Stem Cells and Cancer:** Stem cells serve as a reservoir for generating new cells and can either maintain themselves or differentiate as needed. Uncontrolled cell proliferation from these or other cells can lead to cancer, resulting in tumours that disrupt normal tissue function and may be fatal.

- **Vitamin A's Role in Cell Differentiation and Cancer Prevention:** Retinoic acid, derived from vitamin A, is essential for signalling stem cells to differentiate properly during processes like foetal morphogenesis. High levels of retinoic acid inhibit cell growth, and adequate vitamin A prevents uncontrolled cell proliferation. This regulatory role has made retinoids a focus in cancer risk reduction research.

- **Wnt/β-catenin Signalling and Stem Cell Maintenance:** Retinoids influence cell differentiation through the Wnt/ β-catenin pathway, which is crucial for cell adhesion, tissue growth, development, and maintaining pluripotent stem cell populations. β-catenin prevents stem cells from differentiating, thereby preserving their "stemness."

- **Activation of the Canonical Wnt Pathway:** Wnt proteins activate the canonical Wnt/β-catenin pathway by binding to Frizzled and LRP5/6 receptors on the cell surface. This binding inhibits the destruction complex (comprising Axin, APC, GSK-3β, and CK1), allowing β-catenin to stabilize, accumulate in the cytoplasm, and translocate to the nucleus to regulate gene expression related to cell proliferation and differentiation.

- **ATRA's Mechanism in Modulating β-catenin:** All-trans retinoic acid (ATRA), the active metabolite of Accutane, enhances the activity of the destruction complex by inhibiting the PI3K-AKT pathway. This inhibition promotes GSK-3β-mediated degradation of β-catenin, leading to the differentiation of stem cells and loss of their pluripotent properties.

- **Therapeutic Use of Accutane in Cancer and Effects on Healthy Tissues:** Accutane is utilized in cancer treatment by blocking β-catenin, thereby disrupting the self-renewing capabilities of tumour stem cells and inducing their differentiation. However, ATRA also affects healthy tissues that rely on stem cell populations for maintenance, such as bones, skin, the gut, and the brain, by promoting their differentiation.

3. Natural 'Retinoids' Versus Isotretinoin

As discussed in the previous chapter, the retinoid system is arguably one of the most extensive and significant among the vitamin systems. Consequently, the body meticulously regulates the synthesis of its primary effector, retinoic acid (Vitamin A), through a complex array of negative feedback mechanisms. Excessive retinoic acid signalling can be detrimental, disrupting the growth and development of healthy tissues, particularly in the gut, brain, and musculoskeletal system.

One crucial way the body controls retinoic acid synthesis is by regulating its rate-limiting step through ALDH (aldehyde dehydrogenase) enzymes. However, what occurs when the body is directly exposed to the active metabolite of Vitamin A, all-trans-retinoic acid, bypassing these intermediate regulatory steps? This scenario is precisely what happens during treatment with Accutane. The activity of these enzymes have far-reaching effects, helping to explain enduring changes in vision, dopamine metabolism, and more. In this chapter, I will elucidate the alterations in these enzymes and present the evidence for the lasting adverse effects of retinoic acid.

3.1 Aldehyde Dehydrogenase

Retinoic acid is typically produced in the body through a two-stage process. First, retinol is converted to retinal by enzymes called alcohol/retinol dehydrogenases (ADH/RDH), and then retinal is oxidized to retinoic acid by various ALDH (aldehyde dehydrogenase) enzymes. Aldehyde dehydrogenases represent a large family of enzymes that catalyse the oxidation of aldehydes. This family is diverse, with 19 different isoforms, and plays vital roles in metabolism, the production of neurosteroids, and, relevant to Accutane, the endogenous production of retinoic acid.

$$\text{Retinol} \xrightarrow{\text{RDH}} \text{Retinal} \xrightarrow{\text{ALDH / RALDH}} \text{Retinoic Acid}$$

Vitamin A is classified as a dietary vitamin because the body cannot synthesize it on its own. Toxic levels of vitamin A are also teratogenic, meaning they cause congenital disabilities in developing foetuses. [1] To prevent some of the harmful effects of hypervitaminosis A, the body carefully regulates the enzymes that synthesize retinoic acid through a negative feedback mechanism. These enzymes include aldehyde dehydrogenases (ALDH) and retinaldehyde dehydrogenases (RALDH). [2][3]

One isoform, ALDH2, has been implicated in the phenomenon of "Asian Flush," which is the red facial flushing caused by poor alcohol metabolism, common in some East Asian populations. [4] Although this may seem fairly benign, poor ALDH2 function has been negatively associated with the progression and severity of Alzheimer's disease, given its additional role in the clearance of toxic dopamine metabolites. [5]

Parkinson's disease is characterized by the progressive loss of dopaminergic neurons. Dopamine is a neurotransmitter that governs feelings of satisfaction, pleasure, and excitement, but its primary metabolite, DOPAL, is toxic and can kill dopaminergic cells. This metabolite can be broken down into a less toxic form (DOPAC) by ALDH enzymes. When this process is impaired, it can accelerate the loss of dopaminergic cells, driving the pathogenesis of Parkinson's disease. [6]

$$DOPAL + NAD^+ + H_2O \xrightarrow{\text{ALDH}} DOPAC + NADH + H^+$$

DOPAL is neutralised by ALDH using NAD+ as a cofactor, producing the much less toxic DOPAC.

3.2 Can Accutane be stored in the body?

In order to avoid some of the disastrous effects of hypervitaminosis A, the body carefully regulates the enzymes that synthesise Retinoic Acid (ALDH and RALDH) through a negative feedback mechanism. After excessive exposure to retinoids, it might seem logical to expect a consequent elevation in retinyl esters stored in fatty tissues. Conversely, when the enzyme that stores retinol as retinyl esters (LRAT) is overexpressed, and in this way the body can evade some of the negative effects of high retinol supplementation. [7] Indeed, the primary metabolite of Accutane,

ATRA (all-trans-retinoic acid), induces this enzyme to store retinol as retinyl esters in adipose tissue. [8][9]

$$\text{Retinol} + \text{Fatty Acid} \xrightarrow{\text{LRAT/ARAT}} \text{Retinyl Ester} + \text{Water}$$

In combination with the repression of RALDH/ALDH enzymes and the elevation of LRAT, the body attempts to achieve homeostasis. If this mechanism plays a significant role in humans, it's reasonable to suggest that dietary retinol consumed during Accutane treatment would result in elevated retinyl ester levels in adipose tissue. However, the metabolite of Accutane, all-trans-retinoic acid, cannot itself be directly stored in adipose tissue. [10]

The enzymes that convert stored retinyl esters into usable retinol for circulation are the retinyl ester hydrolases (REHs). A study in mice found that knocking out the lipase HSL (which has REH activity) led to an accumulation of retinyl esters in adipose tissue. Interestingly, these mice also showed a significant reduction in the expression of other key enzymes involved in retinoic acid synthesis, such as ALDH and RALDH1. [11]

$$\text{Retinyl Ester} + H_2O \xrightarrow{\text{REH}} \text{Retinol} + \text{Fatty Acid}$$

Thus, while the metabolite of Accutane, all-trans-retinoic acid, isn't stored in adipose tissue, it could increase liver stores of retinyl esters from dietary sources. This occurs because retinoic acid increases LRAT activity, which is the enzyme that converts retinol into retinyl esters. Furthermore, elevated retinyl ester stores could contribute to other homeostatic processes, such as reducing the expression of key retinoic acid-synthesizing enzymes like ALDH and RALDH.

3.4 β-catenin Regulates ALDH

It turns out that ALDH and the Wnt signalling pathway are closely interconnected, as evidenced by its use as a cancer marker. ALDH is found to be elevated in cancerous tissues, where it is not typically expressed. [12] Not only does elevated ALDH indicate the presence of cancer, but it can also result in a poor response to chemotherapy, as ALDH can protect cancerous stem cells from chemo drugs. [13] However, it is important to note that these are distinct mechanisms. The reason ALDH can be a marker of cancerous growth is related to β-catenin. As previously discussed, β-catenin supports the growth and proliferation of stem cells, including cancerous stem cells.

ALDH is elevated in cancerous tissue precisely because of its capacity to synthesize retinoids. Under normal conditions, elevated ALDH (and related enzymes) would result in increased retinoid synthesis, which would trigger growth arrest and reduced stem cell proliferation. [14] It is only in recent years that scientists have begun to understand this complex feedback loop regulating β-catenin signalling. The increase in retinoid synthesis inhibits β-catenin signalling, leading to differentiation and growth arrest, thereby mitigating the risk of cancer stem cell development. [15]

Under cancerous conditions, however, the tissue does not respond to differentiation, and the elevated β-catenin maintains higher ALDH expression. This overexpression of ALDH can also hinder cancer treatment by neutralizing the toxic effects of chemotherapy drugs. This is why exogenous retinoids, like Accutane, have been found useful in cancer treatment—by inducing differentiation in cancer stem cells through the suppression of β-catenin. [16] Since β-catenin regulates ALDH expression, Accutane treatment leads to a downregulation of ALDH enzymes, resulting in a better response to chemotherapy drugs. [13] Accutane has repeatedly been shown to suppress ALDH activity in this way, enhancing cancer treatments. [17]

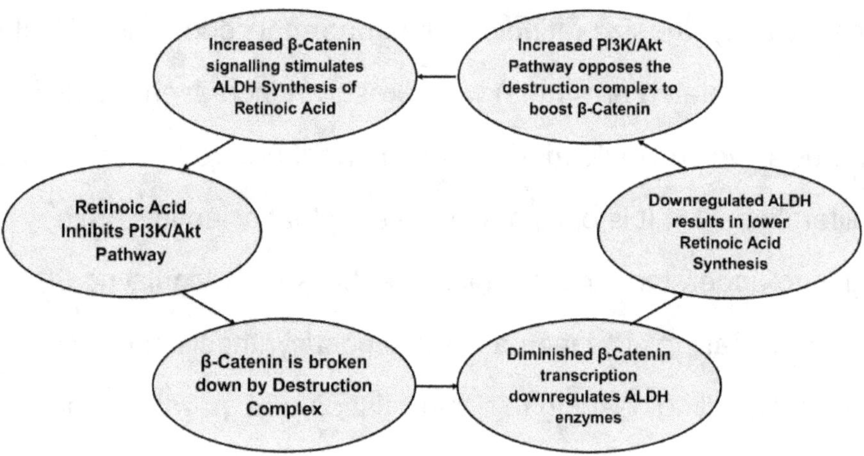

[Fig 6] The negative feedback relationship between ALDH enzymatic activity and β-catenin signalling

3.5 ALDH Can Impact Androgen Signalling

One of the ways of explaining the therapeutic effect of Accutane in treating acne is by modulating androgen signalling. Androgens are the typically male hormones such as Testosterone and DHT (dihydrotestosterone). Several members of the ALDH family more readily bind to androgen substrates than retinol and primarily serve in the production of hormones and neurosteroids. One such isoform is RoHD4 (Retinol dehydrogenase 4), which is prevalent in the skin and liver and acts similarly to 3 alpha-HSD. It catalyses the oxidation of 3α-diol to the much more potent androgen DHT. [18] The presence of this enzyme in the skin might contribute to the development of acne, and the suppression of RoDH4 (via the previously outlined interaction between beta-catenin and ALDH) may constitute one of Accutane's mechanisms of action. [19]

$$3\alpha\text{-diol} \xrightarrow{3\alpha\text{-HSD}/\text{RoDH-4}} \text{Dihydrotestosterone (DHT)}$$

Another product of RoHD4 is androstanedione, which undergoes conversion to DHT in peripheral genital tissue under the action of another enzyme (17b-hydroxysteroid dehydrogenase). [20] The suppressive effect on a number of enzymes sharing both retinoid and steroid dehydrogenase activity has been observed in microarray analysis. 8 weeks of Accutane treatment resulted in a six-fold decrease in 3 beta-HSD expression, which is responsible for the conversion of DHEA into androstenedione. [21] This study also identified a 3-fold suppression 5 alpha-reductase, another key enzyme in the production of DHT.

The impact of Isotretinoin on DHT synthesis could be relevant in understanding the association of the treatment with sexual side effects. The region of the brain best understood to influence sexual desire is the Medial Preoptic Area (MPOA) of the Hypothalamus. It takes inputs from hormonal signals and sensory information to mediate feelings of sexual motivation. Both Estrogen and Androgen Receptors are present in the MPOA and so both Estrogen and DHT can influence copulatory behaviour. By elevating dopamine signalling in the MPOA, DHT can support sexual desire. [22]

In fact, DHT has a variety of unique effects on cognitive function and brain health. Just one example of the specific role of DHT in the brain is that on spatial memory. A battery of cognitive tests on older hypogonadal men treated with either testosterone or DHT found that whilst Testosterone was conducive to verbal memory, only DHT could boost spatial memory. [23] The researchers concluded that role of Testosterone in enhancing verbal memory was through aromatising into Estrogen (E2), based on prior studies in women.

3.6 Conclusion

The body's retinoid metabolism is a delicately balanced system involving enzymes that synthesize, store, and degrade retinoic acid. Aldehyde dehydrogenases (ALDHs), particularly, are pivotal in the natural synthesis of retinoic acid. Importantly however, these enzymes also play significant roles in neurological function and cancer biology. Accutane (isotretinoin), while effective in treating severe acne, introduces substantial disruptions to this balance.

Accutane's primary metabolite, all-trans-retinoic acid (ATRA), could induce the enzyme LRAT to increase the storage of retinol as retinyl esters in adipose tissue. Simultaneously, it represses ALDH and RALDH enzymes, leading to decreased endogenous synthesis of retinoic acid. This dual action may serve as a protective mechanism against hypervitaminosis A but can have unintended consequences. The accumulation of retinyl esters might alter retinoid homeostasis, as well as impairing the other functions of retinoic acid-synthesising enzymes such as ALDH in the brain.

The extent of the suppression of ALDH enzymes by Accutane is evidenced by enhancing the effectiveness of chemotherapy by inhibiting its detoxifying action. Accutane's impact extends beyond dermatology, influencing essential metabolic pathways and enzyme functions. Its ability to disrupt crucial enzymatic processes necessitates a cautious evaluation of its broader physiological implications.

3.7 Chapter Summary

- **Retinoic Acid Production and Regulation:** Retinoic acid is synthesized in two steps—retinol is first converted to retinal by ADH/RDH enzymes, then retinal is oxidized to retinoic acid by ALDH enzymes (19 isoforms). The body regulates retinoic acid levels through ALDH and RALDH enzymes to prevent toxic vitamin A levels.

- **ALDH2 and Neurodegenerative Diseases:** The ALDH2 enzyme metabolizes alcohol, with deficiencies causing "Asian Flush" and increasing Alzheimer's risk by failing to clear toxic dopamine metabolites. Impaired ALDH activity also accelerates the loss of dopaminergic neurons, contributing to Parkinson's disease.

- **Regulation of Retinoic Acid Production:** The body prevents hypervitaminosis A by using a negative feedback mechanism that controls retinoic acid synthesis through ALDH and RALDH enzymes. When retinol levels are high, the enzyme LRAT is overexpressed, converting excess retinol into retinyl esters stored in adipose tissue, a process induced by ATRA.

- **Homeostasis During Retinoid Exposure**: During Accutane treatment, ATRA increases LRAT activity, leading to elevated retinyl ester levels from dietary retinol in fatty tissues. Concurrently, ATRA represses RALDH and ALDH enzymes, helping to maintain vitamin A balance by reducing retinoic acid synthesis.

- **Role of Retinyl Ester Hydrolases (REHs):** REHs convert stored retinyl esters back into retinol for circulation. In mice lacking the REH enzyme HSL, retinyl esters accumulate in adipose tissue and the expression of ALDH and RALDH1 enzymes decreases. This suggests that elevated retinyl esters help suppress retinoic acid production, contributing to overall homeostasis.

- **ALDH as a Cancer Marker and Chemotherapy Resistance:** Elevated ALDH levels are found in cancerous tissues, where they are not typically present. High ALDH activity not only serves as a marker for cancer but also protects cancer stem cells from the effects of chemotherapy, leading to poor treatment responses.

- **Interconnection Between ALDH and β-catenin:** ALDH supports the synthesis of retinoids, which normally would inhibit β-catenin signalling and induce growth arrest. However, in cancerous tissues, the feedback loop is disrupted, allowing β-catenin to maintain high ALDH expression and prevent differentiation, thereby promoting cancer stem cell proliferation.

- **Accutane's Role in Cancer Treatment:** Accutane (ATRA) induces differentiation in cancer stem cells by suppressing β-catenin signalling, which in turn downregulates ALDH enzymes. This suppression enhances the effectiveness of chemotherapy by reducing ALDH-mediated protection of cancer cells, making Accutane a valuable adjunct in cancer therapy.

4. Cell Proliferation in the Brain

Stem cells have become a major focus in biohacking communities, often touted as a potential key to extending youth and health beyond natural limits. However, unchecked cell proliferation also carries risks, notably increasing the chances of cancer and tumour formation. Maintaining a careful balance between stem cell proliferation and differentiation is essential for proper tissue development, while preserving reservoirs of progenitor stem cells to support future tissue repair.

This balance is especially crucial in the brain, which depends on the continuous renewal and proliferation of stem cells for memory formation, learning, and adaptation. The hippocampus, the brain's primary region for memory formation, is particularly relevant to Accutane's neurological effects. Indeed, the hippocampus is a central target in all antidepressant treatments.

Contrary to popular belief, neuroscientists now suggest that inhibited neurogenesis, rather than a mere "chemical imbalance" in the serotonin system, is the primary cause of depression. This raises important questions about the effects of Accutane treatment, particularly since, as previously discussed, retinoids can impair tissue growth and development. In this chapter, I examine evidence showing how retinoic acid disrupts stem cell proliferation in the hippocampus via mechanisms involving beta-catenin.

I further explore the potential of several compounds to restore neurogenesis by enhancing β-catenin signalling, effectively countering the suppressive impact of retinoids. Among these, Lithium stands out for its ability to promote neurogenesis, making it an effective treatment for depression. Additionally, I present compelling evidence on the relationship between retinoids and melatonin, which, like lithium, has significant stem cell proliferative effects. Melatonin interacts extensively with retinoid signalling in the brain, notably by regulating retinoid-synthesising enzymes in the pineal gland and hypothalamus.

4.1 The Hippocampus and Memory Formation

Retinoids exert an anti-proliferative effect on the body. This effect is most strikingly observed in embryos overexposed to vitamin A. If these embryos reach full term, they often suffer from underdeveloped limbs and cleft palates. [1] This explains why Accutane is classified as a teratogen (a substance that disrupts normal foetal development and causes congenital disabilities). It is also the reason for the strict guidelines on birth control for women undergoing Accutane treatment.

However, the anti-proliferative effects of Accutane can also be observed in many adult tissues that rely on pools of stem cells for continual renewal and growth, including the skin, intestines, bone marrow, cornea, hair follicles, and brain (particularly the hippocampus). As discussed throughout this book, retinoids such as Accutane trigger the conversion of these stem cells into specialized cells through differentiation.

In doing so, retinoids maintain a delicate balance between proliferation and differentiation, which is why certain tissues are particularly affected by Accutane treatment. The hippocampus, a region of the brain that relies on stem cells to continue developing new neurons during adulthood, is essential for forming new memories. Accutane significantly inhibits hippocampal neurogenesis, disrupting hippocampal-dependent learning. [2]

Although there is evidence that Accutane may be detrimental to cognitive function, the results are sometimes mixed. For instance, when rats were treated with Accutane prior to a two-stage maze task in which both stages were identical, it was found that Accutane impaired explicit memory during the second stage. [3] However, one month after Accutane exposure ended, explicit memory was recovered. This finding was supported by a study in mice that similarly showed a disruption in learning a radial maze task. [4]

Crandall et al. (2004) demonstrated that after 42 days of treatment with retinoic acid, hippocampal cell proliferation had almost halved. From this, they concluded that the decline in memory was directly related to Accutane's impact on neurogenesis. Nonetheless, when rats were maintained on a long-term vitamin A-deficient diet, they also suffered from deficits in memory and hippocampal neurogenesis. This suggests that retinoic acid signalling must be delicately balanced, as both excessive and insufficient levels can damage memory formation. [5]

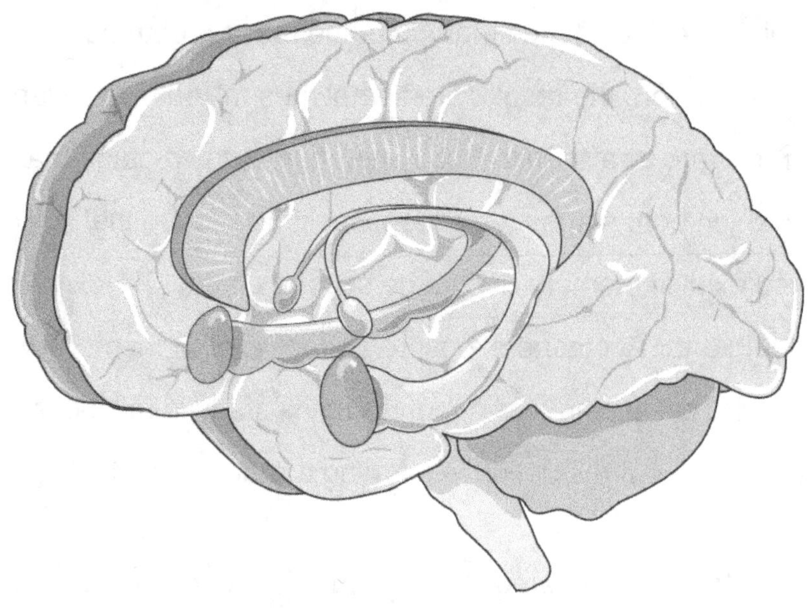

[Fig 7] **Image of the two hippocampi in each hemisphere of the brain highlighted as the two curved red and green structures**. (Brain – hippocampus, Servier Medical Art is licensed under CC BY 4.0 https://smart.servier.com/smart_image/hippocampus/)

4.2 β-catenin is Needed for Brain Health

As previously established, β-catenin signalling is essential for maintaining stem cell populations in many tissues that undergo continual growth and repair throughout adulthood. The brain, particularly the hippocampus, is one such region. The hippocampus is critical for the generation of episodic and spatial memory. Neuroplasticity in the hippocampus is necessary to form new memories throughout adulthood.

It has been found that when β-catenin is ablated in hippocampal cell cultures, synaptic strength diminishes. Neurons lacking β-catenin become thin and spindly, with a reduced amplitude of spontaneous glutamatergic currents. [6] Conversely, enhancing β-catenin signalling in transgenic mice led to greater neuronal growth and even enlarged brains due to an increase in neural stem cell populations. [7] Understanding the role of β-catenin is key to explaining the evidence that Accutane inhibits new cell growth in the hippocampus. [8]

Notably, the neurological role of β-catenin is not confined to the hippocampus, as it also greatly impacts synaptic activity in two other regions: the hypothalamus and the amygdala. The hypothalamus is a part of the limbic system that controls the release of hormones involved in diverse processes, including sexual responses, hunger, and circadian rhythms. Hypothalamic cells are also subject to both growth and regulation by β-catenin, which can be influenced by oestradiol, a hormone that activates the PI3K/Akt pathway.

Importantly, the action of oestradiol is the exact opposite of the mechanism by which Accutane suppresses β-catenin. The significance of oestradiol is especially relevant for women due to the oestrous cycle and the periodic changes it induces in synaptic structures. [9] Given this evidence, it is perhaps unsurprising that hypothalamic cells (along with hippocampal cells) are among the neuronal cells most vulnerable to apoptosis (cell death) in response to retinoic acid exposure. [10]

Another structure within the limbic system is the amygdala, which consists of two clusters of nuclei in the centre of the brain and plays a pivotal role in regulating memory, emotional response, and feelings of reward and pleasure. Like the hypothalamus, the amygdala is also significantly influenced by β-catenin.

There is evidence that β-catenin is required for transferring newly formed memories into long-term memory, and specific deletion of β-catenin prevents this memory consolidation. [11] Furthermore, researchers have been able to induce dysregulation of the amygdala in rats by applying retinoic acid, which resulted in heightened fear and anxiety responses.

4.3 Lithium Enhances Hippocampal Neurogenesis

Lithium is a trace metal found in tap water at low doses, as well as in some foods such as cereals, potatoes, cabbage, and tomatoes. [12] While it is typically thought of as a medication for psychosis and mania, lithium actually offers a range of positive effects on brain health, including enhancing brain-derived neurotrophic factor (BDNF) and reducing oxidative stress. [13] Although lithium is still stigmatized as a potent 'zombifier,' suppressing cognition and mood, this couldn't be further from the truth. A 2009 meta-analysis found that healthy subjects treated with lithium experienced no adverse effects on any of the tested cognitive domains, and only minor effects on patients with affective disorders. [14]

Much of lithium's brain-boosting effects can be attributed to its action on the Wnt/β-catenin pathway. Lithium has been found to increase cytoplasmic levels of β-catenin, essentially having the opposite effect of Accutane. Lithium acts as an agonist of the canonical Wnt signalling pathway by inhibiting GSK3-β activity, thereby releasing β-catenin from the destruction complex. [15] This leads to the typical β-catenin proliferation effects, particularly relevant in the brain, where it induces neurogenesis in the hippocampus.

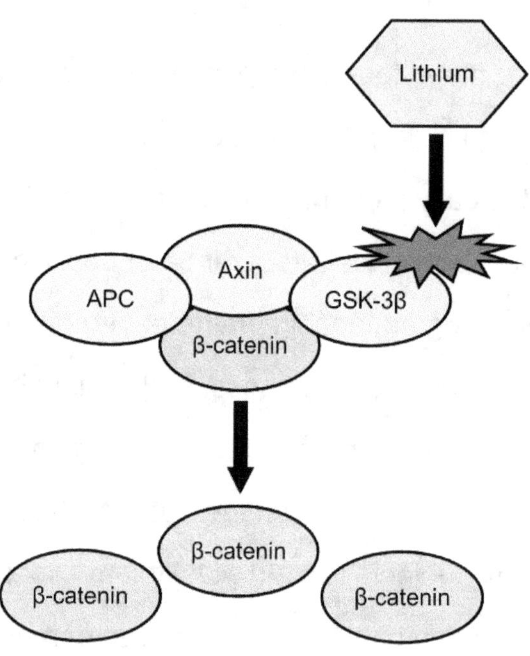

[Fig 8] **Lithium inhibits GSK3-β, releasing β-catenin from the destruction complex.**

In fact, neuroimaging has demonstrated that lithium accumulation in the hippocampus is responsible for the larger hippocampal volumes observed in patients being treated for bipolar disorder. Chronic high-dose lithium treatment in human hippocampal cultures increases the generation of progenitor cells, neuroblasts, and neurons. [16] The proliferative effect of lithium on hippocampal cells is the mirror opposite of Accutane's effect.

Lithium potently induces neurogenesis; Hellweg et al. found that lithium increases NGF (nerve growth factor) in the frontal cortex (+23%), hippocampus (+72%), amygdala (+74%), and limbic forebrain (+47%). [17] Given that the leading theory of depression involves a lack of neurogenesis, the possible implications of Accutane inhibiting β-catenin should be clear. Conversely, lithium appears to promote neurogenesis through the direct opposite effect of Accutane on β-catenin.

Whilst Lithium is perhaps the best attested medication for enhancing β-catenin signalling in the brain (and elsewhere), it isn't the only substance known for doing so. In fact, two other chemicals naturally synthesised in the body also appear to potently induce β-catenin: Butyrate and Melatonin. Butyrate exists in small quantities in certain foods but is also a major product of the gut microbiota, produced in colon via the fermentation of dietary fibres. Melatonin is the body's 'Sleep Hormone' released from the pineal gland at night. Melatonin especially has an interesting interaction with the β-catenin as it appears to be intimately interconnected with Retinoic acid pathway in the brain, which will be explored throughout the rest of this chapter.

4.5 The Hypothalamus and Melatonin

The circadian rhythm is the 24-hour cycle that determines changes in behaviour over the day and night. This process governs the sleep-wake cycle and is influenced by environmental cues such as light exposure. The biological functions regulated by the circadian rhythm are broad, including eating habits, digestion, body temperature, and importantly – hormones.

The hypothalamus is a small structure in the limbic system that plays a very powerful role in synchronising the circadian rhythm. The primary signal used by the body to control the circadian rhythm comes from the photoreceptors, which are cells within the retina responsible for vision. Photoreceptors provide vital environmental information to the hypothalamus to ensure appropriate hormonal secretion.

Of all the roles of Vitamin A, perhaps the best attested is maintenance of eye health. Loss of night vision and drying of the cornea are both symptoms of prolonged Vitamin A deficiency. [18] Unsurprisingly, alterations to the eyes and vision are also common complaints during Accutane treatment. One such troubling side effect is the complete loss of night vision in some patients. [19] The cause of this symptom has been found to be inhibition of the enzyme 11cRDH (11-cis-retinol dehydrogenase). [20] This results in lower levels of 11-cis-retinal, a vital constituent of photoreceptors in the retina. [21]

It is concerning that there's even a suggestion that night blindness resulting from Accutane treatment can be permanent. [22] Given how fundamental photoreceptors are to the circadian rhythm, some researchers have hypothesised that these changes could underlie a hormonal effect via the hypothalamus. The suprachiasmatic nucleus (SCN) is the circadian centre within the hypothalamus. The SCN then informs the pineal gland to secrete the hormone melatonin in response to the daily changes in photoreception.

Furthermore, the retina-hypothalamic-pineal axis controls reproductive behaviour through changes in hormone secretion from the pituitary gland. These signals inform the gonads to produce hormones such as testosterone. Disrupting photoreception could therefore have a downstream impact on androgen status. [23]

The pineal gland is a small structure directly in the centre of the brain. Whilst many fantastical claims are made about the significance of the pineal gland, even at one point believed to be the "seat of the soul", it does in fact play a crucial role in the secretion of melatonin. This is the sleep hormone that is secreted at night, and thereby synchronises the sleep-wake cycle. The role of vitamin A in the circadian rhythm is consolidated by evidence that retinoic acid and melatonin apparently have an antagonistic (opposing) relationship. [24]

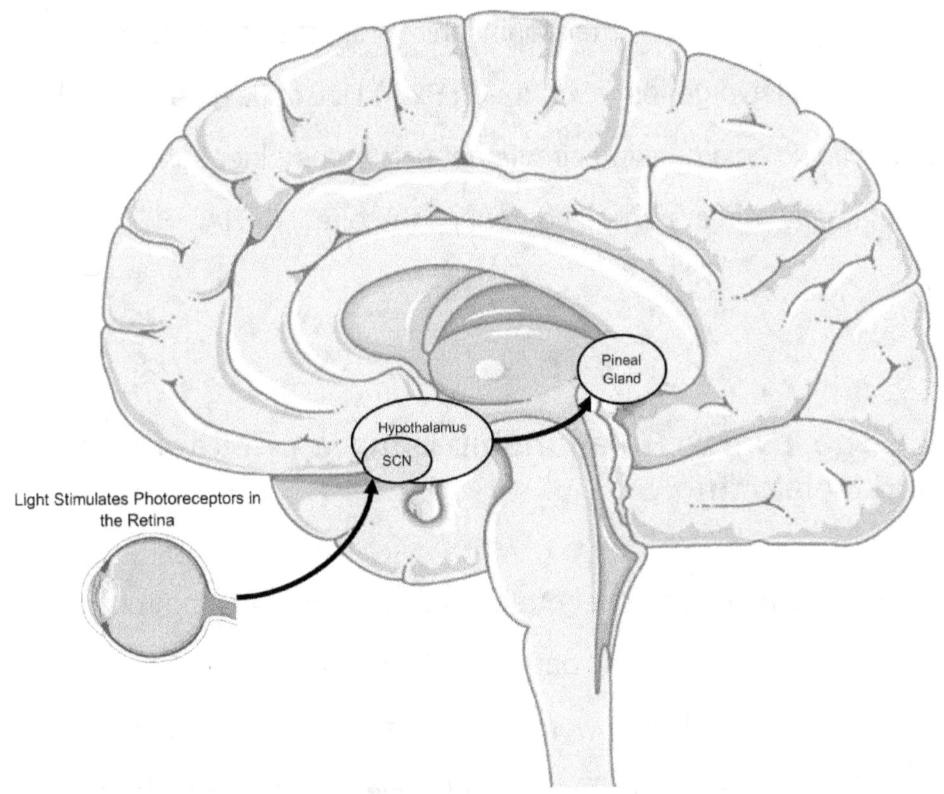

[Fig 9] **A simplified model of the Retinohypothalamic axis**, (Altered from the original to show Retinohypothalamic axis/Servier Medical Art is licensed under CC BY 4.0 https://smart.servier.com/smart_image/brain-sagittal/ https://smart.servier.com/smart_image/eye-cataract-stage-1/)

There are diurnal (circadian) changes in the expression of genes in the pineal gland needed for the synthesis of retinoic acid. [25] Retinoic acid synthesis in the pineal gland increases during the night, when melatonin is being produced. However, when administered together, melatonin inhibits expression of retinoic acid-responsive genes (such as CYP26A1). So, despite melatonin and retinoic acid peaking simultaneously in the pineal gland at night, melatonin apparently dampens the effect of RA.

4.6 The Inverse Relationship Between Retinoic Acid and Melatonin

A study on the effects of shorter days (short photoperiod) on retinoic acid found that all pathways linked to retinoids, from synthesis to breakdown, were repressed by a shorter interval of light. The cause of this effect was identified as increased levels of melatonin. [26] Treatment with melatonin mimicked the effect of short photoperiod in suppressing genes regulated by retinoic acid in the hypothalamus. Nightly injections of melatonin into the hypothalamus also reduced the activity of enzymes involved in synthesising retinoic acid, such as Raldh1.

These findings confirm that the synthesis of RA in the hypothalamus is controlled by melatonin. Changes in the hypothalamus itself are a probable candidate for the depression-related behaviours caused by Accutane treatment. There is in vitro evidence that isotretinoin induces cell death in GT1-7 hypothalamic cell cultures. [27]

One set of genes that also appear to be diurnally regulated in the hypothalamus are those involved in Wnt/β-catenin signalling. I have written extensively on the significance of β-catenin in understanding the impact of isotretinoin on cell proliferation. One of the proteins that has an inhibitory effect on β-catenin signalling is DKK3. Like the genes involved in RA synthesis, DKK3 is also increased during long photoperiods. β-catenin is strongly implicated in neurogenesis, making it key for understanding the neurological effects of Accutane more broadly. [28]

The evidence presented so far shows that light exposure (photoperiod) influences the expression of genes involved in the synthesis of retinoic acid in the hypothalamus, and this is an effect mediated by melatonin secretion from the pineal gland. Not only do the diurnal changes in melatonin secretion appear to have an inhibitory effect on retinoic acid synthesis, but exogenous administration also dampens the effect of RA on gene expression.

Photoperiod could also influence the secretion of hormones via signalling from the hypothalamus to the pituitary gland. For this reason, changes in photoreception are important for seasonal mating. The increase in mating behaviours of livestock during the transition to autumn, with shorter light periods, is reliant upon neurogenesis in the hypothalamus. The higher levels of cell proliferation in the hypothalamus with decreasing day length are a consequence of increased melatonin from the pineal gland. [29]

Melatonin has repeatedly been shown to increase cell proliferation in several regions of the brain, including the hippocampus and ventral midbrain. [30] This is in stark contrast to the effect of isotretinoin in these same regions, which instead suppresses hippocampal neurogenesis. [31] In fact, the most striking evidence for the diverging effects of melatonin and isotretinoin is the case reports where melatonin even induces acne in some patients. [32]

As previously stated, many of isotretinoin's biological effects can be understood in terms of repression of β-catenin signalling, and the subsequent reduction in stem cell proliferation. With this in mind, another interesting point of conflict is found with respect to hair growth. Melatonin increases the viability of dermal papilla cells, the cells that generate hair follicles, enhancing β-catenin. [33] Hair loss is a known side effect of Accutane treatment, although the exact mechanisms involved haven't been clearly identified. [34]

The positive effect of melatonin on hair growth is curious, as melatonin has also been found to increase 5-alpha-reductase activity, a principal driver of androgenic alopecia. [35][36] Isotretinoin exerts a suppressive effect on 5-alpha-reductase, which could also constitute one of its anti-acne mechanisms.

4.8 Butyrate and Cell Proliferation in the Gut

As previously detailed, many organs rely on the maintenance of a progenitor pool of stem cells throughout adulthood, which are vital for tissue repair, regeneration, and normal organ functioning. One tissue that relies on progenitor cells in this way is the intestine, and this process is partially regulated by a short-chain fatty acid called butyrate. Butyrate is endogenously produced through microbial fermentation of dietary fibres in the lower intestinal tract. Short-chain fatty acids (SCFAs) such as acetate, propionate, and butyrate are produced by the bacteria in the colon from starch and dietary fibres. Some fermented foods, such as Parmesan or Pecorino cheeses, contain very small quantities of butyrate naturally, and anyone familiar with the supplement sodium butyrate will recognise its distinctly cheesy odour.

The primary function of SCFAs is in energy metabolism, where they provide up to 70% of the energy requirement of the epithelial cells that line the colon. Although butyrate only constitutes 15% of endogenous SCFAs in the colon, it is arguably the most important, capable of exerting profound effects throughout the body. [37]

A 2011 case-control study found that ulcerative colitis (UC) was strongly associated with prior isotretinoin exposure, with a 4.4 times greater risk compared to controls. [38] Ulcerative colitis is a chronic inflammatory condition of the colon, with primary symptoms of abdominal pain and diarrhoea. During flare-ups, symptoms may include eye irritation, painful joints, and even bone degradation. The risk of developing UC dramatically increased with isotretinoin dose, with each additional 20 mg per day associated with a 1.5-fold increase in the odds ratio.

The FDA's MedWatch has also reported 83 cases of newly developed Inflammatory Bowel Disease (IBD) following exposure to isotretinoin. [39] The average latency period in one study was found to be around three years. Using the Bradford Hill criteria, which consider temporality as a measure of causation, the researchers were able to dismiss any association—a decision that has come under some criticism. [38][40]

In the absence of β-catenin signalling, stem cells undergo rapid differentiation, and the progenitor stem cell pool becomes depleted. This was most plainly demonstrated in a 2023 study on mice, where researchers performed a β-catenin gene ablation on adult mice and observed the effects on the intestinal tract. [41] The loss of β-catenin triggered the intestinal stem cell population to terminally differentiate, resulting in the loss of function and ultimately death. This represents an exaggerated mechanism of action similar to that of Accutane, which suppresses β-catenin through HOXA5 induction, resulting in the loss of intestinal stem cells. [42]

A case report of a 17-year-old who developed Inflammatory Bowel Disease (IBD) following isotretinoin treatment even posited inhibition of epithelial cell growth as a potential cause. [43] Conversely, agents that activate the Wnt pathway to enhance β-catenin, such as lithium, have been found to increase intestinal stem cell populations. [44][45]

Butyrate, like lithium (or other β-catenin inducers, e.g., valproate), can support the renewal of stem cell populations. Butyrate also shares some of the same epigenetic effects as these β-catenin inducers by inhibiting histone deacetylases (HDACs) and thus increasing gene transcription by maintaining an open chromatin structure. Interestingly, activation of the Wnt/β-catenin pathway appears to be linked to HDAC inhibition. [46]

Studies have found that butyrate, at the right concentration, can support the self-renewal of human embryonic stem cells (ESCs). [47] Conversely, very high and very low concentrations of butyrate could trigger differentiation in ESCs. The researchers identified butyrate's demethylating and HDAC-inhibiting action to be responsible for its impacts on stem cells, and these effects could be partially mimicked by typical HDAC-inhibiting medications such as valproate. [48]

Notably, many of the same transcription factors butyrate relies on for its stem cell-renewing effects, such as c-Myc, Oct4, and Sox2, are all targeted for suppression by Accutane. It's important to recognise that the relationship between butyrate and β-catenin is complex and has confounded researchers for years, even being referred to as the "butyrate paradox." Whilst butyrate is able to enhance epithelial and colonocyte proliferation, it's also able to inhibit the proliferation of cancerous stem cells on account of a differential effect on β-catenin-TCF complexing. [49] Overall, the benefits of butyrate within the β-catenin model predominate.

4.7 Conclusion

In conclusion, Accutane exerts a profound anti-proliferative effects on the body by altering the balance between stem cell proliferation and differentiation. Its mechanism of action involves promoting the differentiation of stem cells into specialized cells, thereby reducing the pool of stem cells necessary for tissue renewal and growth. This effect is particularly evident in embryos overexposed to vitamin A derivatives, leading to severe congenital disabilities such as underdeveloped limbs and cleft palates. Consequently, Accutane is classified as a teratogen, necessitating strict birth control measures for women undergoing treatment.

In adults, Accutane's impact extends to various tissues reliant on stem cell populations, including the skin, intestines, bone marrow, cornea, hair follicles, and notably, the brain's hippocampus. By inhibiting Wnt/β-catenin signalling—a pathway crucial for maintaining stem cell populations—Accutane significantly reduces hippocampal neurogenesis. This suppression can disrupt hippocampal-dependent learning and memory formation, with studies showing mixed results on cognitive function and some indicating reversible effects post-treatment.

Accutane also affects other brain regions such as the hypothalamus and amygdala, which play vital roles in hormonal regulation, emotional responses, and memory consolidation. The medication's interference with β-catenin signalling in these areas may contribute to heightened fear, anxiety responses, and hormonal imbalances.

Moreover, Accutane can impair photoreceptor function in the retina by inhibiting the enzyme 11cRDH, pointing to similar effects within the hypothalamus. This impairment may disrupt the circadian rhythm, and downstream hormonal processes regulated by the hypothalamus and pineal gland, affecting sleep patterns and reproductive hormones.

Contrastingly, substances like lithium, melatonin and butyrate have been shown to enhance β-catenin signalling and promote neurogenesis. Lithium increases hippocampal neurogenesis and has neuroprotective effects without significant adverse cognitive outcomes. Melatonin, which regulates circadian rhythms, also promotes cell proliferation and opposes some of the effects of retinoic acid.

4.8 Chapter Summary

- **Impact on Neurogenesis and Memory:** Accutane reduces hippocampal neurogenesis, impairing memory and learning. Cognitive deficits may recover after treatment, but both excessive and insufficient retinoic acid disrupt memory formation.

- **Balance of Retinoic Acid Signalling:** Retinoids regulate the balance between cell proliferation and differentiation. Proper retinoic acid levels are essential for tissue maintenance and cognitive function, as both high and low levels can cause adverse effects.

- **Critical Role of β-catenin in the Hippocampus:** β-catenin signalling is essential for maintaining neural stem cells in the hippocampus, supporting synaptic strength, neuronal growth, and the formation of episodic and spatial memories. Loss of β-catenin impairs neuron structure and function, while increased signalling promotes brain growth and stem cell proliferation.

- **Impact on Hypothalamus and Amygdala Function:** β-catenin also regulates synaptic activity in the hypothalamus and amygdala, influencing hormone release, emotional responses, and memory consolidation. Disruption of β-catenin by retinoic acid leads to heightened fear, anxiety, and increased vulnerability of these neuronal cells to apoptosis.

- **Accutane's Suppression of β-catenin and Neurological Effects:** Accutane inhibits β-catenin signalling, counteracting oestradiol's activation of the PI3K/Akt pathway. This suppression reduces neurogenesis in the hippocampus, impairs memory and learning, and makes hypothalamic and hippocampal cells more susceptible to cell death, thereby affecting cognitive and emotional functions.

- **Lithium Enhances Brain Health:** Found in tap water and foods like cereals and potatoes, lithium boosts brain health by increasing brain-derived neurotrophic factor (BDNF) and reducing oxidative stress without adversely affecting cognition in healthy individuals or those with mood disorders.

- **Activation of Wnt/β-catenin Pathway:** Lithium acts as an agonist of the canonical Wnt/β-catenin pathway by inhibiting GSK3-β, which increases β-catenin levels. This promotes neurogenesis in the hippocampus, leading to larger hippocampal volumes and increased generation of neurons and progenitor cells.

- **Photoreceptors and Hypothalamus Regulate Circadian Rhythm:** The circadian rhythm, a 24-hour cycle governing sleep-wake patterns and various biological functions, relies on environmental cues like light exposure. Photoreceptors in the retina send signals to the hypothalamus, specifically the suprachiasmatic nucleus (SCN), to synchronize these rhythms.

- **Vitamin A's Role in Eye Health and Accutane's Effects:** Vitamin A is essential for eye health, with deficiencies leading to night blindness and corneal dryness. Accutane treatment can cause similar visual side effects by inhibiting the enzyme 11cRDH, reducing levels of 11-cis-retinal necessary for photoreceptor function, potentially resulting in permanent night blindness.

- **Antagonistic Relationship Between Retinoic Acid and Melatonin:** The pineal gland increases retinoic acid synthesis at night when melatonin is produced. However, melatonin inhibits the expression of retinoic acid-responsive genes like CYP26A1, indicating an antagonistic relationship that plays a role in circadian regulation.

- **Melatonin Suppresses Retinoic Acid Synthesis in the Hypothalamus:** Increased melatonin levels, whether due to shorter daylight periods or direct administration, repress genes involved in retinoic acid (RA) synthesis, such as Raldh1, in the hypothalamus.

- **Contrasting Effects on Neurogenesis:** Melatonin promotes cell proliferation and neurogenesis in brain regions like the hippocampus and ventral midbrain, enhancing β-catenin signalling. In contrast, isotretinoin (Accutane) suppresses β-catenin signalling and neurogenesis in these regions, which may explain some of its neurological side effects.

- **Influence on Hair Growth:** Melatonin increases the viability of dermal papilla cells and enhances β-catenin signalling, promoting hair growth. Accutane, however, may cause hair loss due to its repression of β-catenin signalling, although the exact mechanisms are not fully understood.

- **Butyrate's Role in Intestinal Health:** Butyrate, a short-chain fatty acid produced by gut bacteria fermenting dietary fibres, is crucial for maintaining the progenitor pool of intestinal stem cells, which are vital for tissue repair, regeneration, and normal organ functioning.

- **Association Between Isotretinoin (Accutane) and Ulcerative Colitis:** Some studies, including a 2011 case-control study, have found a strong association between isotretinoin exposure and an increased risk of developing ulcerative colitis (UC), with higher doses correlating with greater risk.

- **β-catenin Signalling and Intestinal Stem Cells:** β-catenin signalling is essential for the maintenance of intestinal stem cells. Suppression of this pathway, as observed with isotretinoin treatment, can lead to rapid differentiation and depletion of these stem cells, potentially resulting in impaired intestinal function and conditions like inflammatory bowel disease (IBD).

- **Butyrate's Protective Effects and the "Butyrate Paradox":** Butyrate can support the renewal of stem cell populations by inhibiting histone deacetylases (HDACs) and activating β-catenin signalling. While it promotes the proliferation of normal epithelial and colonocyte cells, it can inhibit the proliferation of cancerous stem cells—a phenomenon known as the "butyrate paradox." This complex relationship underscores butyrate's overall beneficial role within the β-catenin model.

5. Dopamine Transmission and Receptors

Throughout this book, it becomes clear that retinoids can profoundly influence tissue differentiation and enzymatic activity, particularly that of ALDH. These combined effects are crucial for understanding how Accutane may impact the dopaminergic system. Dopamine is a vital neurotransmitter, essential for regulating feelings of reward, excitement, and motivation. Dysregulation of dopamine can lead to depression, mania, and even psychosis—all outcomes documented in research on Accutane's neurological effects.

Among Accutane's neurological impacts, disruptions to dopamine are particularly relevant for understanding the reported symptoms of depression and low mood. However, this system remains enigmatic, and neuroscientists have yet to reach a consensus on why retinoid-synthesising enzymes are so frequently co-expressed with dopamine pathways in the brain.

Research in this area of neuroscience is limited, so much of this chapter is based on my own hypotheses, developed using the best available scientific literature. Evidence suggests that Accutane may lead to lasting changes in dopaminergic system function, not only through epigenetic modifications of retinoid-synthesising enzymes but also by altering gene expression of the D2 dopamine receptor.

5.1 Accutane Impacts Dopamine Transmission Through ALDH

There is abundant evidence pointing to Accutane treatment causing lasting repression of ALDH in various contexts. One of the most frequently observed effects is night blindness. The specific isoform of ALDH responsible for maintaining photoreceptors in the retina is 11cRDH (11-cis-retinol Dehydrogenase). By repressing this enzyme through the mechanism outlined above, Accutane can cause lasting changes in vision under low-light conditions. [1][2]

However, given the diverse roles of ALDH enzymes, the range of possible consequences is extensive. The detoxifying function of ALDH is particularly relevant, as it breaks down reactive aldehydes in response to various drugs and pollutants. For example, ALDH2 is responsible for oxidizing acetaldehyde into the much less harmful acetic acid. Another, perhaps less appreciated role of ALDH, is detoxifying harmful byproducts of dopamine transmission in the brain. The metabolites of dopamine, such as DOPAL, are neurotoxic, and excessive dopamine can result in the death of dopaminergic neurons. However, another member of the ALDH family, RALDH1, metabolizes these destructive aldehydes, thereby protecting dopaminergic neurons. [3]

Given the involvement of ALDH in neurodegenerative diseases, it should be concerning that administering retinoic acid causes the repression of these enzymes. [4] 'Asian Flush' may seem like a minor issue, but underactivity of ALDH2 is negatively associated with the progression of Alzheimer's and Parkinson's diseases. Parkinson's disease is characterized by the progressive loss of dopaminergic neurons, driven by dopamine metabolites such as DOPAL. [5][6]

A useful analogy in understanding the neurological effects of ALDH repression is Disulfiram, a medication used to treat alcoholism by inhibiting ALDH2. It was long believed that Disulfiram made alcohol consumption less rewarding by triggering the accumulation of toxic aldehydes, similar to the mechanism behind 'Asian Flush.' However, research has since shown that it curbs addictive behaviour by directly impacting dopamine transmission.

By preventing the clearance of toxic dopamine metabolites, Disulfiram treatment results in lower levels of extracellular dopamine. [7] This makes Disulfiram effective in treating addiction to other substances unrelated to alcohol, such as amphetamines. [8] It is therefore unsurprising that patients treated with Disulfiram often report muted feelings of reward. Given the evidence suggesting that retinoic acid has a similar effect on ALDH in certain contexts, Disulfiram could provide insight into some of the side effects of Accutane treatment.

5.2 D2 Dopamine receptor

In addition to impacting dopamine transmission by disrupting key enzymes, Accutane also appears to directly influence gene transcription for dopamine receptors. There are five subtypes of dopamine receptors in the brain, each with different distributions and effects. These subtypes can be divided into two families: the D1-like family and the D2-like family. The D1-like family receptors are G-protein Gsα-coupled, meaning they mediate stimulatory effects, such as increased heart rate and other fight-or-flight responses.

The D2-like family receptors are Giα-coupled, meaning they inhibit the formation of cAMP. These D2 receptors can be further subdivided into autoreceptors and heteroreceptors. The autoreceptor mediates a negative feedback response to dopamine. In contrast, the heteroreceptor is located on postsynaptic sites, where its binding mediates the classical effects of dopamine as a neurotransmitter.

As previously mentioned, the D2 dopamine receptor is inhibitory, meaning that binding to it can result in lower neuronal excitability by exerting a hyperpolarizing effect. This is because these receptors are coupled to Gi/o proteins, which inhibit calcium channels and activate inwardly rectifying potassium channels. When D2 receptors are present on the presynaptic neuron, they exert a negative feedback effect, leading to lower dopamine transmission. [9] Activation of the D2-autoreceptor triggers behaviours typically associated with reduced dopamine signalling, such as decreased exploratory locomotion and a loss of motivation for stimulants like amphetamine.

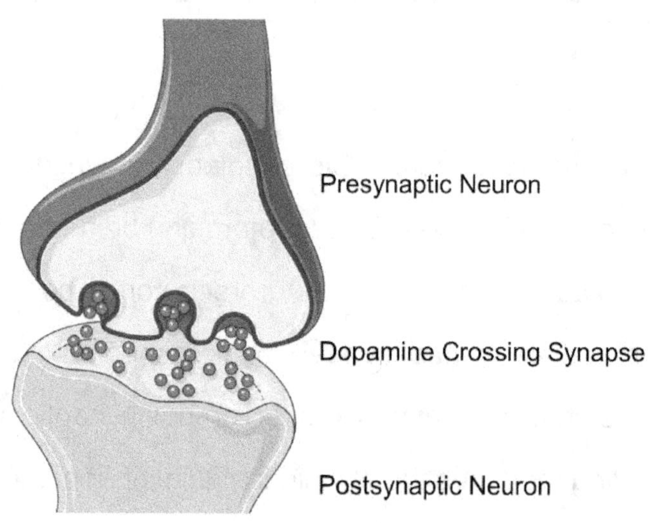

[Fig 10] **Transmission of dopamine across synaptic cleft from Presynaptic to Postsynaptic Neuron,** (Servier Medical Art is licensed under CC BY 4.0 https://smart.servier.com/smart_image/smart-synapse-ov/)

Conditional knockout of either the D2 heteroreceptor or autoreceptor has shown that the loss of the autoreceptor results in heightened dopamine responses. [10] These animals became 'super sensitive' to stimulants such as cocaine and exhibited hyperactivity. This finding is corroborated by evidence that lower midbrain D2 autoreceptors are found in individuals with a stronger drive for novelty seeking, owing to increased dopaminergic release. [11]

Splicing of the mRNA encoding the D2 receptor has revealed both short and long forms, with the long form believed to be the D2-heteroreceptor and the short form thought to be the D2-autoreceptor (although both may have autoreceptor activity).

5.3 Retinoic Acid and Dopamine Receptor Gene Expression

Now that the details of the D2 receptor have been explored, I can present the evidence for the possible disruption caused by Accutane. As explained at length in previous articles, Accutane can be understood as a differentiating agent—that is, forcing pluripotent (stem) cells to become differentiated (specialized) cells. This trait is particularly useful in treating many cancers that maintain pluripotency and undergo continual cell proliferation, forming tumours. In these cases, retinoids can trigger these cells to differentiate, thereby robbing cancerous cells of their pluripotent nature.

One common example often cited is neuroblastoma cells, which differentiate into D2 dopaminergic neurons in response to Accutane. Intriguingly, these cells are induced more strongly into the short variant than the long variant. This suggests that Accutane may preferentially induce the expression of autoreceptors rather than heteroreceptors. [12]

Accutane can influence the behaviour of the D2 receptor because it contains a RARE (retinoic acid response element). The effect of increasing D2 autoreceptor expression relative to the heteroreceptor would, therefore, paradoxically hamper dopamine transmission, rather than enhance it. This could help explain the association between Accutane treatment and depressive symptoms, which are characteristic of reduced dopamine activity.

However, a complete absence of retinoic acid can also have harmful effects on dopamine neuron differentiation, which a failure to properly develop either D2 autoreceptor or heteroreceptors. In fact, animal studies have shown this to be the case with Retinoic Acid receptor knockout mice developing a phenotype similar to Parkinsons. It's evident that both too much and too little retinoic acid, especially during development, can have disastrous consequences for the dopaminergic system in particular. [21]

5.4 Boosting ALDH Activity With ALCAR

The dopaminergic system is deeply complex, and few interventions are considered free from side effects. While dopamine is crucial for mediating feelings of pleasure and reward, improper dopamine signalling is implicated in psychosis. [13] Despite the widespread use of amphetamines in the treatment of ADHD, even prescription medications can cause oxidative stress and inflammation. [14][15] Any direct intervention in dopamine signalling is best avoided. However, ALDH can be effectively targeted with certain medications and over-the-counter supplements. One such supplement that shows promise in this regard is Acetyl-L-Carnitine (ALCAR).

ALCAR is simply the acetylated form of the naturally occurring L-carnitine. Studies indicate that ALCAR can reduce Parkinson's symptoms and protect the brain against the neurotoxic effects of amphetamines. There are several mechanisms underlying

ALCAR's antioxidant properties, including free radical scavenging. [16] One significant finding is that ALCAR, along with another antioxidant, CoQ10, appears to potently upregulate ALDH activity in the brain. [17]

ALCAR with CoQ10 lowered the levels of malondialdehyde (MDA) and pro-inflammatory cytokines in the cerebellum of rats treated with propionic acid. Propionic acid significantly downregulated ALDH1A1, and treatment with ALCAR (alone and with CoQ10) effectively restored its activity compared to controls. The dosage used in this study was relatively high compared to most over-the-counter supplements, equivalent to approximately 1.2g for a 70kg human.

Another study on ALCAR in reversing Parkinson's in rats found similar dosing to be effective in protecting dopaminergic neurons. This study induced Parkinson's via injections of a toxic dopamine metabolite, 6-hydroxydopamine (6-OHDA). The researchers even attributed ALCAR's neuroprotective effects to the activation of the Wnt/β-catenin pathway. Inhibiting GSK3-β had the opposite effect on β-catenin compared to retinoic acid. [18] Even higher doses of 3g daily in humans have been found to be well-tolerated and effective in peripheral nerve regeneration. [19] Other studies have pointed to the tolerability of higher ALCAR doses (>2g daily), particularly in the context of neurodegenerative disorders. [20]

5.5 Conclusion

In conclusion, Accutane exerts significant effects on aldehyde dehydrogenase (ALDH) enzymes. One of the most well-known consequences is night blindness due to the repression of 11cRDH, an ALDH isoform crucial for photoreceptor function in low-light conditions. Concerningly, this enzyme suppression can result in lasting visual impairments.

The role of ALDH enzymes extends to detoxifying harmful aldehydes, including neurotoxic dopamine metabolites like DOPAL. Repression of ALDH by Accutane raises concerns about neurodegenerative risks, as impaired detoxification can lead to the death of dopaminergic neurons—a hallmark of conditions such as Parkinson's disease. The analogy with Disulfiram, an ALDH2 inhibitor used in treating alcoholism, illustrates how inhibiting ALDH can affect dopamine transmission and reduce feelings of reward, paralleling some of the mood alterations reported with Accutane use.

Accutane also appears to influence dopamine receptor gene transcription, particularly affecting the D2 receptors. By potentially increasing the expression of D2 autoreceptors over heteroreceptors, Accutane may decrease dopamine transmission, contributing to depressive symptoms and reduced motivation. There is a delicate balance required in retinoic acid levels, as both excess and deficiency can adversely impact the dopaminergic system. Research into protective measures like Acetyl-L-Carnitine (ALCAR) shows promise in upregulating ALDH activity and offering neuroprotective effects, particularly in the context of dopamine and excitotoxicity.

5.6 Chapter Summary

- **Night Blindness Due to ALDH Repression:** Accutane represses the ALDH enzyme 11cRDH in the retina, leading to night blindness by impairing the maintenance of photoreceptors under low-light conditions.

- **Impaired Detoxification of Aldehydes:** Accutane's repression of various ALDH enzymes disrupts the detoxification of reactive aldehydes and dopamine metabolites like DOPAL, increasing neurotoxicity and the risk of dopaminergic neuron death.

- **Increased Risk of Neurodegenerative Diseases:** Reduced activity of ALDH2 from Accutane treatment is associated with the progression of Alzheimer's and Parkinson's diseases, as impaired ALDH function hinders the clearance of toxic substances in the brain.

- **Similarity to Disulfiram's Effects on Dopamine:** Like Disulfiram, which inhibits ALDH2 and affects dopamine transmission to curb addictive behaviours, Accutane's repression of ALDH may lead to altered dopamine levels and muted feelings of reward, contributing to some of its neurological side effects.

- **Roles of D2-like Receptors:** D2-like receptors inhibit the formation of cAMP and are subdivided into autoreceptors and heteroreceptors. Autoreceptors provide negative feedback on dopamine release from presynaptic neurons, while heteroreceptors are located on postsynaptic sites, mediating dopamine's classical neurotransmitter effects.

- **Behavioural Effects of D2 Autoreceptor Activity:** Activation of D2-autoreceptors leads to decreased neuronal excitability and dopamine transmission, resulting in behaviours associated with reduced dopamine signalling, such as decreased exploratory movement and diminished motivation for stimulants like amphetamine.

- **Consequences of D2 Autoreceptor Loss:** Conditional knockout studies show that losing D2-autoreceptors causes heightened dopamine responses, making animals hypersensitive to stimulants like cocaine and increasing hyperactivity. This is linked to increased dopaminergic release and a stronger drive for novelty seeking. The D2 receptor exists in short (likely the autoreceptor) and long (likely the heteroreceptor) mRNA splice forms.

- **Accutane Induces Differentiation of Stem Cells:** Accutane acts as a differentiating agent that forces pluripotent stem cells, including cancerous cells like neuroblastomas, to become specialized cells such as D2 dopaminergic neurons. This reduces their ability to proliferate and form tumours.

- **Preferential Expression of D2 Autoreceptors:** Accutane influences the D2 dopamine receptor gene, which contains a retinoic acid response element (RARE), leading to increased expression of the D2 autoreceptor (short variant) over the heteroreceptor (long variant). This shift hampers dopamine transmission by enhancing negative feedback, potentially contributing to depressive symptoms associated with reduced dopamine activity.

- **Need for Balanced Retinoic Acid Levels:** Both excessive and insufficient retinoic acid can disrupt dopamine neuron differentiation and function. Animal studies show that lack of retinoic acid receptors leads to Parkinson's-like symptoms, indicating that proper retinoic acid signalling is crucial for maintaining a healthy dopaminergic system.

- **Acetyl-L-Carnitine (ALCAR) Targets ALDH to Support Dopamine Function:** ALCAR, the acetylated form of L-carnitine, has been shown to reduce Parkinson's symptoms and protect the brain from the neurotoxic effects of amphetamines by upregulating aldehyde dehydrogenase (ALDH) activity and acting as an antioxidant.

- **ALCAR Combined with CoQ10 Enhances Neuroprotection:** Studies indicate that ALCAR, especially when combined with Coenzyme Q10 (CoQ10), lowers levels of malondialdehyde (MDA) and pro-inflammatory cytokines in the brain. This combination effectively restores ALDH1A1 activity in animal models, suggesting a potent neuroprotective effect.

- **Effective Dosing and Activation of Wnt/β-catenin Pathway:** Higher doses of ALCAR are well-tolerated. The neuroprotective benefits include the activation of the Wnt/β-catenin pathway, offering potential therapeutic effects for neurodegenerative disorders.

6. Serotonin: The 5-HT1A Receptor

6.1 The 5-HT1A Receptor

The 5-HT1A receptor is a serotonin receptor, meaning it is bound by the neurotransmitter serotonin to exert its effects. Serotonin has long been associated with "happiness," stemming from early scientific evidence that serotonin depletion leads to depressive symptoms. The vast majority of antidepressant medications work on this neurotransmitter and are called SSRIs (Selective Serotonin Reuptake Inhibitors).

The 5-HT1A receptors are inhibitory receptors because they are G-protein-coupled. When bound, they reduce AMPA-evoked currents. AMPA receptors are responsible for fast synaptic transmission, so by binding to the 5-HT1A receptor, neuronal activity is suppressed.

The receptor is subdivided into two types, with different distributions in the brain: autoreceptors and heteroreceptors. The autoreceptors are localized within the brainstem in a structure called the Raphe

Nuclei. This structure, located in the middle of the brain, is the origin of all other serotonergic neurons that project outward.

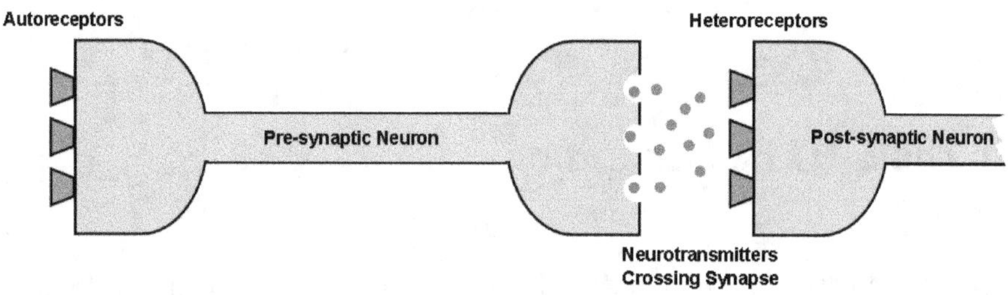

As the name suggests, the (presynaptic) autoreceptor serves to self-regulate serotonin transmission throughout the brain via a negative feedback mechanism. When serotonin accumulates within the Raphe Nuclei, it binds to these receptors to limit further serotonin release (since 5-HT1A receptors are inhibitory). Because autoreceptors have a self-limiting effect on serotonin transmission, overexpression limits serotonin release to other areas of the brain. This overexpression has also been notably identified in autopsies of patients with depression. [1]

The postsynaptic heteroreceptor sites are distributed in the limbic and cortical regions. The limbic system is responsible for regulating emotion, learning, and sexual behaviour. Like the autoreceptor, binding at the 5-HT1A heteroreceptor triggers hyperpolarization of the neuron, reducing its firing rate. The heteroreceptors are found on two different types of neurons with opposing effects: interneurons and pyramidal neurons.

Interneurons are GABAergic, meaning they release the inhibitory neurotransmitter GABA. [2] Conversely, pyramidal neurons release the excitatory neurotransmitter glutamate and are particularly abundant in the cerebral cortex. These pyramidal neurons play a key role in memory, learning, and attention, and are opposed by the GABAergic interneurons that regulate their activity.

The differing behavioural effects of binding at the heteroreceptor versus the autoreceptor were most clearly demonstrated by Garcia-Garcia et al. in their 2017 study. They took different groups of mice and knocked out (removed) either heteroreceptors or autoreceptors.

They found that mice lacking heteroreceptors displayed depressive symptoms characteristic of anhedonia, rather than anxiety. Conversely, mice with ablated autoreceptors experienced heightened anxiety but still displayed a drive for reward. [2] This study provides insight into how the 5-HT1A receptor influences sexual behaviour, with binding at the heteroreceptor being particularly relevant. Supporting this idea is the fact that the medication Flibanserin, used to treat hypoactive sexual desire disorder, binds most potently to heteroreceptor sites. [3]

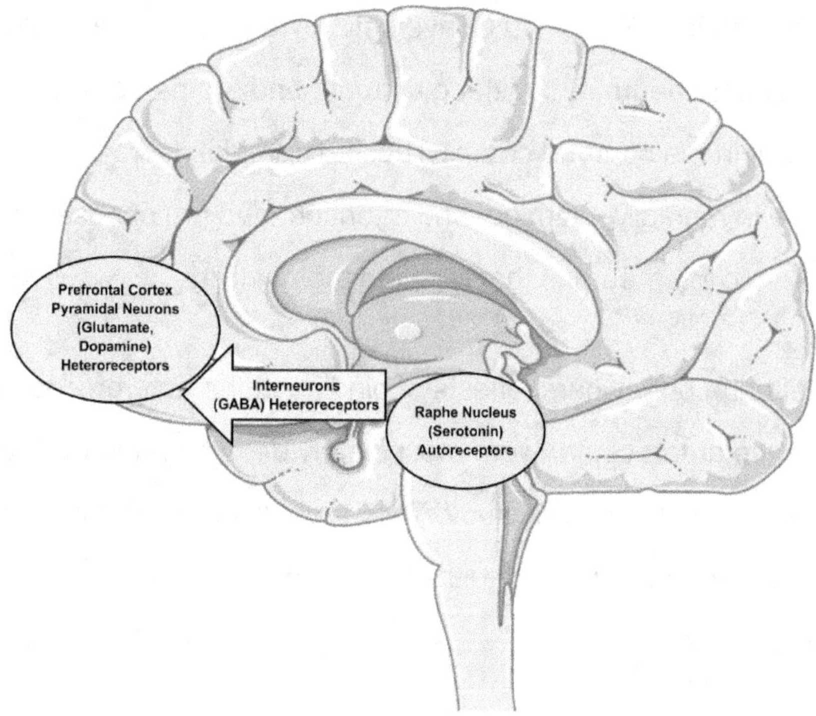

[Fig 11] **The 5-HT1A Circuitry from the Raphe Nucleus to the Prefrontal Cortex**. (Servier Medical Art is licensed under CC BY 4.0, Sagittal Graphic, Servier / Modified from original image with added graphics to indicate 5-HT1A Circuitry)

6.2 Isotretinoin Increases 5-HT1A Autoreceptor Protein

Now that I have provided a general mechanistic overview of the 5-HT1A receptor, I can present the evidence for how it is impacted by Isotretinoin treatment. Reilly et al. exposed cell lines from the Raphe Nuclei to Isotretinoin and observed a massive increase in 5-HT1A autoreceptor protein levels. After just 48 hours of exposure, there was up to a 70% increase in autoreceptor protein. [4] The authors of the study suggest that this is a significant factor in the depressive behaviour exhibited by people treated with the acne drug.

In line with the behaviour of the autoreceptor previously outlined, an increase in autoreceptor levels would inhibit serotonin release to the rest of the brain, particularly to the 5-HT1A heteroreceptor sites. Under activation of the heteroreceptor could induce some of the same anhedonic symptoms observed in the Garcia-Garcia study.

A crucial regulator of 5-HT1A expression is the transcription factor Deaf1, which has a dual effect of inhibiting autoreceptor expression while enhancing heteroreceptor expression. Deaf1 expression is regulated by the PI3K/Akt pathway, which is also influenced by

Isotretinoin. Isotretinoin disrupts this pathway, resulting in elevated GSK3β levels. Since GSK3β inactivates Deaf1 through phosphorylation, this could explain the significant increase in autoreceptor protein levels induced by Isotretinoin. This effect of Isotretinoin is contrasted against that of Lithium, which has the opposite action on GSK3β. For this reason, Lithium can boost the expression of the post-synaptic heteroreceptor 5-HT1A while repressing the autoreceptor. [5]

6.3 Conclusion

Accutane (isotretinoin) significantly impacts the serotonergic system by altering the expression and function of 5-HT1A serotonin receptors. Specifically, isotretinoin increases the levels of 5-HT1A autoreceptors in the Raphe Nuclei—a brain region crucial for regulating serotonin release throughout the brain via negative feedback mechanisms. This overexpression leads to reduced serotonin availability in limbic and cortical regions, where 5-HT1A heteroreceptors play key roles in emotion, learning, and sexual behaviour.

The under activation of heteroreceptors due to decreased serotonin levels can result in depressive symptoms characterized by anhedonia, as evidenced by studies showing that mice lacking these receptors exhibit such behaviours. This mechanism provides a plausible explanation for the depressive symptoms reported by some patients undergoing Accutane treatment.

At the molecular level, isotretinoin disrupts the PI3K/Akt pathway, leading to elevated levels of GSK3β. This enzyme inactivates the transcription factor DEAF1, which normally inhibits autoreceptor expression while enhancing heteroreceptor expression. The inactivation of DEAF1 results in increased autoreceptor levels and decreased heteroreceptor activity, further exacerbating serotonin imbalance. This contrasts with the action of lithium, which inhibits GSK3β and thereby promotes DEAF1 activity, leading to a healthier balance between autoreceptors and heteroreceptors.

6.4 Chapter Summary

- **Function and Significance of 5-HT1A Receptors:** The 5-HT1A receptor is a serotonin receptor involved in mood regulation, with serotonin depletion leading to depressive symptoms. Most antidepressants are SSRIs that target serotonin to alleviate these symptoms.

- **Types and Locations of 5-HT1A Receptors:** These inhibitory receptors are divided into autoreceptors and heteroreceptors. Autoreceptors are located in the Raphe Nuclei of the brainstem and regulate serotonin release via negative feedback. Heteroreceptors are found in limbic and cortical regions and reduce neuronal firing when activated.

- **Role in Depression and Anxiety:** Overexpression of autoreceptors limits serotonin release to other brain areas and has been observed in patients with depression. Studies show that mice lacking heteroreceptors exhibit depressive symptoms like anhedonia, while mice lacking autoreceptors display increased anxiety but maintain motivation for rewards.

- **Influence on Sexual Behaviour and Therapeutic Applications:** Binding at heteroreceptors affects sexual behaviour, with medications like Flibanserin—used to treat hypoactive sexual desire disorder—binding potently to these sites, highlighting the therapeutic relevance of 5-HT1A heteroreceptors.

- **Isotretinoin Increases 5-HT1A Autoreceptor Levels:** Reilly et al. exposed Raphe Nuclei cell lines to isotretinoin and observed up to a 70% increase in 5-HT1A autoreceptor protein levels within 48 hours, potentially contributing to depressive symptoms in treated individuals.

- **Elevated Autoreceptors Inhibit Serotonin Release:** Increased autoreceptor levels inhibit serotonin release to the rest of the brain, particularly affecting 5-HT1A heteroreceptor sites, which may lead to anhedonic symptoms similar to those observed when heteroreceptor activity is under activated.

- **Disruption of Deaf1 Regulation via PI3K/Akt Pathway:** Isotretinoin disrupts the PI3K/Akt pathway, leading to elevated GSK3β levels that inactivate Deaf1, a transcription factor that normally inhibits autoreceptor expression and enhances heteroreceptor expression. This disruption may explain the significant increase in autoreceptor protein levels induced by isotretinoin.

7. The Prefrontal Cortex

The frontal cortex is the most highly developed area of the human brain compared to other animals, responsible for advanced cognitive functions, motivation, reward processing, and delayed gratification. Evidence suggesting that Accutane treatment significantly influences this critical region is therefore concerning. A notable 2005 brain imaging study by Bremner et al. found that treatment with Accutane reduced activity in this area of the brain. The authors could only hypothesise about the underlying reasons for this change and its potential longevity.

In this chapter, I present evidence that Accutane may alter the circuitry of the prefrontal cortex by influencing the differentiation pattern of a key set of neurons known as interneurons. These neurons regulate prefrontal cortex activity by releasing the inhibitory neurotransmitter GABA. Retinoic acid appears capable of altering neural progenitor cell differentiation, potentially leading to lasting changes in prefrontal cortex function.

7.1 Evidence from brain imaging studies

Of all the evidence for Accutane's troubling effects on the brain, the most damning comes from a 2005 study by Bremner et al. In this study, PET scans were performed on 28 men and women to compare changes in brain metabolism following either four months of Accutane or antibiotic treatment. The results were shocking: the Isotretinoin group experienced a 21% decrease in activity in the orbitofrontal cortex, compared to a 2% increase in the antibiotic group. [1]

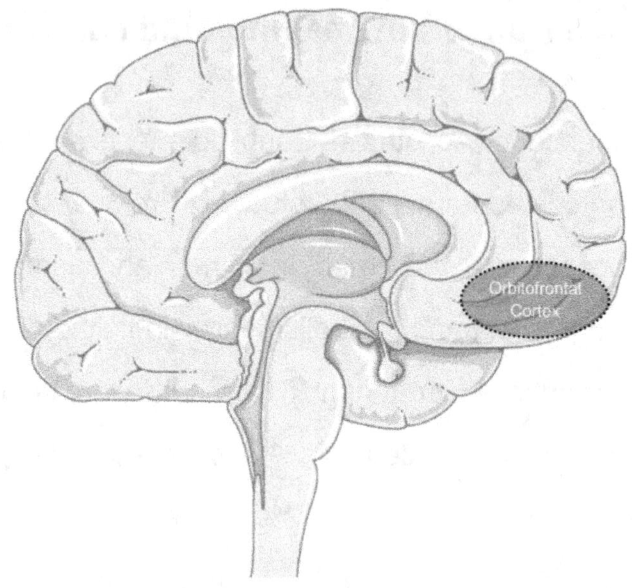

[Fig 12] **Image of Brain modified with label to indicate approximate location of Orbitofrontal Cortex** (modified with label of Orbitofrontal Cortex,Servier Medical Art is licensed under CC BY 4.0 https://smart.servier.com/smart_image/brain-sagittal/)

The orbitofrontal cortex is a region within the prefrontal cortex involved in higher cognitive functions, such as reward-based decision-making. This finding strongly supports the link between depressive symptoms and prior Accutane use. The researchers also identified an intriguing connection between reports of headaches during treatment and the relative degree of suppression of brain metabolism, with those reporting more severe headaches also showing greater reductions in orbitofrontal cortex activity.

The orbitofrontal cortex (OFC) evaluates decisions and choices based on expected rewards and punishments. For this reason, abnormalities in OFC activity can be linked to disorders of reward perception, such as obsessive-compulsive behaviour or hypersexuality. [2] Damage to the prefrontal cortex often leaves individuals unable to consider the long-term consequences of decision-making, resulting in choices that prioritize immediate gratification. [3] Functional neuroimaging has found that the orbitofrontal cortex is one of the brain regions most implicated in depression. Patients with depression were found to have a 32% smaller orbitofrontal cortex compared to controls. [4]

7.2 The Neuroanatomical Basis for Reduced Orbitofrontal Activity

While retinoic acid is highly relevant to neuronal differentiation in embryonic tissues, in adulthood, RA-synthesizing enzymes are restricted to cortical regions – particularly those involved in executive functioning. [5] This narrow band of the cortex is characterized by the presence of RALDH3, with slower maturation compared to surrounding cortical tissue. The finding that four months of isotretinoin treatment reduces the activity of the orbitofrontal cortex, therefore, has a strong neuroanatomical basis. [6] The fact that this region has slower maturation compared to surrounding cortical areas supports the role of retinoic acid signalling during adulthood. Opposing the action of CYP26b1 is ALDH1A3, which is present in the superficial layer of the prefrontal cortex and is involved in synthesizing RA.

The findings by Bremner et al. are clearly troubling for anyone treated with the acne medication, but do they have a neuroanatomical basis? As it turns out, the enzyme that metabolizes retinoic acid, CYP26b1, is present in the interneurons that govern the activity of the prefrontal cortex. [7] These interneurons connect the thalamus and the prefrontal cortex, and CYP26b1's role in regulating retinoic acid synthesis may help explain the changes in orbitofrontal activity in Accutane patients. By knocking out the CYP26b1 enzyme, researchers can mimic the effects of overexposure to retinoic acid. Mice with the CYP26b1 enzyme knocked out display a dramatic increase in parvalbumin (PV) expressing interneurons.

These interneurons are GABAergic, meaning they release the inhibitory neurotransmitter GABA. [8] GABA is the primary inhibitory neurotransmitter in the central nervous system and binds to GABA-A and GABA-B receptors. Binding to GABA-A receptors results in hyperpolarization of the neuron, making it harder to reach the threshold required for an action potential and subsequently reducing that neuron's firing rate. Many of the excitatory neurons present in the prefrontal cortex, such as pyramidal neurons, are regulated by PV interneurons, with GABA inhibiting excitation. [9]

Some studies have used Muscimol, a GABA agonist, as a method to investigate the function of these neurons. These studies suggest that activation of PV neurons worsens working memory. [10] It's possible that elevated RA signalling during isotretinoin treatment could force the differentiation of NSCs into PV-expressing interneurons, thereby increasing inhibitory action on the prefrontal cortex—evidenced by the decrease in activity in the orbitofrontal cortex. [11]

Whether the decrease in orbitofrontal cortex metabolism following isotretinoin treatment is a direct effect or secondary to its impact on the hippocampus is difficult to determine. This is because there are input and output connections between the orbitofrontal cortex and hippocampus, and in particular, the ventral hippocampus is important for dopamine innervation in the medial prefrontal cortex. [12]

7.3 Retinoic Acid Increases GABAergic Interneurons

A 2011 study by Chatzi et al. further supported the role of retinoic acid in the differentiation of embryonic stem cells into GABAergic interneurons. Furthermore, they found that retinoic acid is required to activate the enzyme that converts glutamate into GABA. [13] In RALDH3 knockout mice, lateral ganglionic eminence progenitor cells fail to differentiate into GABAergic interneurons. [14]

The most insightful work in elucidating the relationship between retinoic acid and GABAergic interneurons was performed by Huang et al. (2020). The researchers found that rats chronically exposed to retinoic acid displayed depressive behaviour, which coincided with changes in neural excitability and plasticity. In the hippocampus, there was an increase in the expression of GABA receptors, along with a simultaneous decrease in glutamate receptors. [15] In fact, not only was there an increase in GABA receptors, but also an upregulation of the glutamate decarboxylase enzyme, which synthesizes GABA from glutamate. The net effect was a range of depressive-like behaviours, indicated by decreased sucrose preference and increased immobility in the tail suspension test.

Huang et al. further analysed the input-output relationship of excitatory postsynaptic potential and population spikes in the hippocampus of rats exposed to retinoic acid. They found that the population spike amplitude of the retinoic acid-treated rats was significantly smaller than that of the vehicle group, supporting the notion that retinoic acid decreases neuronal excitability in the dentate gyrus. The population spike is a sudden change in voltage from pyramidal neurons, often considered a marker of synaptic plasticity, such as long-term potentiation needed for memory formation.

To further explore the role of GABA in these changes in neural excitability, the researchers performed quantitative real-time PCR. Markers for GABA were significantly elevated in the hippocampus, along with a decrease in mRNA expression of glutamate. Similar increases in GABA receptor mRNA were observed in the prefrontal cortex and hypothalamus of RA-exposed rats. The most profound changes in mRNA were found in the GABRB3 gene encoding for the GABA-A receptor in the prefrontal cortex, GABRA2 in the hypothalamus, and GABRA3 in the hippocampus.

Quantitative PCR analysis by Takayama et al. (2014) found GABRA3 to be a retinoic acid response gene. [16] In the hippocampus, there was a decrease in mRNA expression for two of the AMPA receptor subunits, GluR1 and GluR3, suggesting a dysregulation of glutamate signalling. Given the importance of glutamate in synaptic plasticity, these changes could also underlie learning impairments. Reduced GluR1 expression also occurs in aging brains and is a known risk factor for Alzheimer's disease. [17]

7.4 Conclusion

Accutane has been repeatedly demonstrated to cause profound disruption to cognitive function. This is best evidenced by a 2005 study by Bremner et al. which found a substantial 21% decrease in activity within the orbitofrontal cortex of patients undergoing Accutane treatment – an effect not seen in those treated with antibiotics. The orbitofrontal cortex is critical for reward-based decision-making and emotional regulation. The activity in this very significant region of the prefrontal cortex relies on a delicate balance between excitatory and inhibitory signals, in particular mediated by GABAergic interneurons. Accutane appears to disrupt this balance by influencing the differentiation and activity of GABAergic interneurons. Specifically, increased retinoic acid levels can lead to the overexpression of parvalbumin-expressing interneurons. This results in enhanced inhibitory GABAergic signalling, which reduces neuronal excitability in the prefrontal cortex and may contribute to depressive symptoms.

Further studies corroborate these findings, demonstrating that chronic exposure to retinoic acid elevates GABA receptor expression while decreasing glutamate receptor levels in the hippocampus and prefrontal cortex. Such alterations impair synaptic plasticity and neural excitability, leading to deficits in learning, memory, and mood regulation. The observed decrease in glutamate receptors like GluR1 also aligns with known risk factors for neurodegenerative conditions such as Alzheimer's disease. Collectively, these findings suggest that Accutane's impact on neurotransmitter systems and neuronal differentiation can lead to significant neuropsychiatric side effects.

7.5 Chapter Summary

- **Accutane Significantly Reduces Orbitofrontal Cortex Activity:** A 2005 study by Bremner et al. found that patients treated with Accutane experienced a 21% decrease in activity in the orbitofrontal cortex (OFC), compared to a 2% increase in those treated with antibiotics. This reduction supports a link between Accutane use and depressive symptoms.

- **Orbitofrontal Cortex Role in Decision-Making and Mood Disorders:** The OFC is involved in reward-based decision-making and evaluating consequences. Abnormalities in this region are associated with disorders like depression, obsessive-compulsive behaviour, and hypersexuality. Damage to the OFC can lead to impulsive choices focused on immediate gratification.

- **Retinoic Acid's Role in the Adult Cortex and Isotretinoin's Impact:** In adults, retinoic acid (RA)-synthesizing enzymes like RALDH3 are restricted to cortical regions involved in executive functions, such as the orbitofrontal cortex. Isotretinoin treatment reduces activity in this region, which is significant due to the slower maturation of these areas and the role of RA signalling in their development.

- **CYP26b1 Enzyme and Parvalbumin Interneurons:** The enzyme CYP26b1, which metabolizes RA, is present in interneurons that regulate prefrontal cortex activity by connecting the thalamus and prefrontal cortex. Knocking out CYP26b1 mimics RA overexposure and leads to an increase in parvalbumin (PV) expressing GABAergic interneurons, which inhibit neuronal firing.

- **Inhibition of Prefrontal Cortex Activity by PV Interneurons:** PV interneurons release GABA, the primary inhibitory neurotransmitter that hyperpolarizes neurons and reduces their firing rate. This increased inhibitory action affects excitatory neurons like pyramidal neurons in the prefrontal cortex, potentially worsening working memory and reducing orbitofrontal cortex activity.

- **Uncertain Direct or Indirect Effects on Orbitofrontal Cortex Metabolism:** It is unclear whether the decrease in orbitofrontal cortex metabolism from isotretinoin treatment is a direct effect or secondary to its impact on the hippocampus. The orbitofrontal cortex and hippocampus are interconnected, with the ventral hippocampus playing a crucial role in dopamine innervation of the medial prefrontal cortex.

- **Retinoic Acid Promotes Differentiation into GABAergic Interneurons:** Studies by Chatzi et al. (2011) demonstrated that retinoic acid (RA) is essential for the differentiation of embryonic stem cells into GABAergic interneurons by activating the enzyme that converts glutamate into GABA. Mice lacking the enzyme RALDH3 fail to produce these interneurons.

- **Chronic RA Exposure Leads to Depressive Behaviours and Altered Neurochemistry:** Huang et al. (2020) found that rats chronically exposed to retinoic acid exhibited depressive-like behaviours, such as decreased sucrose preference and increased immobility. This was associated with increased expression of GABA receptors and glutamate decarboxylase in the hippocampus, along with decreased expression of glutamate receptors.

- **Reduced Neuronal Excitability and Synaptic Plasticity:** Electrophysiological analyses showed that RA-treated rats had significantly smaller population spike amplitudes in the hippocampus, indicating decreased neuronal excitability in the dentate gyrus. This reduction may impair synaptic plasticity necessary for memory formation.

- **Altered Gene Expression May Underlie Learning Impairments:** Quantitative PCR revealed elevated markers for GABA and increased GABA receptor mRNA (notably GABRB3, GABRA2, and GABRA3) in various brain regions, alongside decreased mRNA expression of AMPA receptor subunits GluR1 and GluR3. These changes suggest dysregulated glutamate signalling, which could contribute to learning impairments and are associated with risks for Alzheimer's disease.

8. PPARs: Dopamine and Endocannabinoids

Peroxisome Proliferator-Activated Receptors (PPARs) are a fascinating group of receptors involved in lipid metabolism, cell proliferation, and differentiation. Their pivotal role in metabolic processes has long made them a valuable target for treating conditions like diabetes. PPARs are also one of the targets of retinoic acid, through which Accutane can affect various metabolic activities. A lesser-known function of these receptors is their role in the brain, where they appear to influence neurotransmitter behaviour and the activity of certain neurosteroids.

PPARs are also involved in sebum production, making them particularly relevant for understanding how Accutane's effects may extend throughout the body, including to the eyes, where they may play a role in the development of Meibomian Gland Dysfunction. In this chapter, I explore this evidence and discuss the potential impact of Accutane treatment on the brain, drawing on insights from the scientific literature.

8.1 What are PPARs?

Peroxisome Proliferator-Activated Receptors (PPARs) are a group of nuclear receptor proteins that function as transcription factors to regulate metabolic health. There are three types of PPARs: alpha, gamma, and delta. When bound by fatty acids and their derivatives (such as prostaglandins), PPARs influence processes such as fat burning, lipid storage, and glucose metabolism. [1] PPAR-alpha serves to metabolise fatty acids, increasing the beneficial HDL cholesterol while decreasing triglycerides. [2] PPAR-gamma is the target of medications that boost insulin sensitivity in type 2 diabetes by promoting the storage of fatty acids in adipocytes, thus correcting dyslipidaemia. [3] These medications, called thiazolidinediones, shift the body's metabolism towards using glucose as the main fuel substrate rather than free fatty acids. [4]

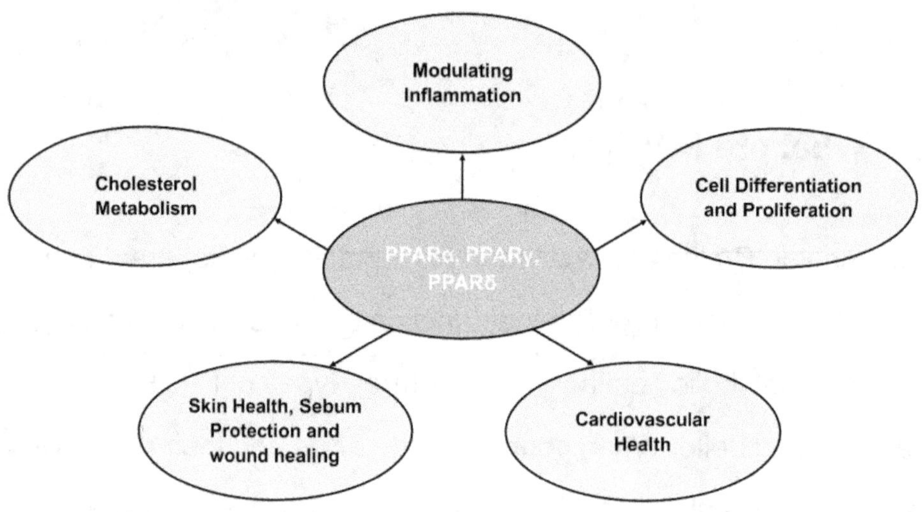

[Fig 13] The diverse roles of PPARs throughout the body.

Among the many side effects of Accutane, elevation of LDL cholesterol and triglycerides is of immediate concern. This may put even young patients at risk of developing cardiovascular disease and atherosclerosis, so practitioners often require frequent blood tests. [5] [6] The regulation of lipids by PPAR is not confined to the liver and adipose tissue but also occurs within the sebaceous glands. The sebaceous lipids, which can be exploited by bacteria in the development of acne, are regulated by PPAR and its interaction with androgens and growth factors. It's clear that the relationship between Accutane and PPAR is key to understanding both how it so effectively treats acne while also incurring such adverse health effects.

8.2 What's the Evidence for Accutane Impacting PPARs?

The evidence for the relationship between Accutane and PPARs is complex and occasionally contradictory. It's established that agonists for PPARs, such as thiazolidinediones or fibrates, enhance sebum production. [7] This has made PPARs of particular interest not only in the context of metabolic conditions such as diabetes, but also in severe cystic acne. Given how radically Accutane impacts metabolic health, it's not surprising that there's plenty of evidence indicating that it has a suppressive effect on PPAR signalling. Patients treated with Accutane are often required to undergo regular monitoring of their cholesterol levels, as both cholesterol and triglycerides can spike in response to the medication, posing a significant increase in the risk of developing cardiovascular disease. [8]

Typically, this state of dyslipidaemia leads to lower sensitivity to insulin, and thus leads to greater levels of circulating insulin. This would seem to be counterproductive for an acne medication, as insulin insensitivity is a known cause of acne, and the greater levels of insulin and IGF-1 (Insulin-like Growth Factor-1) that occur during puberty are considered to be the main triggers of acne during this period of growth. Nonetheless, meta-analyses don't identify a significant change in insulin sensitivity in response to Accutane despite the heightened risk of developing dyslipidaemia. [9][10] While there's even some evidence that Accutane might increase insulin sensitivity,[11] there's also evidence for reduced insulin sensitivity. [12]

Perhaps the clearest evidence for Accutane's impact on PPAR signalling comes from a study on Meibomian Gland Dysfunction (MGD), a dry eye disease. Dry eyes are a frequent complaint by those treated with the acne drug, and an investigation into its pathogenesis identified a marked decrease in the function of PPAR-gamma. As previously stated, PPARs aren't just involved in lipogenesis within the body, but also in the sebaceous glands. [13] The Meibomian glands are essentially large specialized sebaceous glands, and suppression of PPAR-gamma results in reduced lipid secretion. This leaves the aqueous layer of the eye vulnerable to evaporation.

However, in other contexts, isotretinoin has been found to enhance PPAR-gamma expression. This is understandable, as PPARs form a heterodimer with Retinoid X Receptor, a target receptor of retinoids. In adipose tissue, PPAR-gamma mRNA is increased early in isotretinoin treatment. The key determiner in the direction of effect is likely the length of treatment and dosing, with short-term increases in PPAR-gamma and insulin sensitivity, which are eventually followed by a decline. [14]

Given the somewhat contradictory evidence surrounding PPAR and Accutane, a better understanding could be gathered from indirect evidence. One of the functions of PPAR-gamma is to facilitate retinoic acid signalling by regulating enzymes involved in its production. In particular, PPAR-gamma activation enhances RDH10 and RALDH2. [15] I've previously detailed the evidence for Accutane suppressing the retinoic acid synthesizing enzymes in a negative feedback loop. [16] One notable example is that suppression of retinoid synthesizing enzymes can lead to lasting night-blindness following treatment with the acne drug. [17] In this way, it could be inferred that suppression of PPAR might represent a feedback mechanism in response to excessive retinoid signalling.

8.3 β-catenin Regulates PPAR

One of the regulators of PPAR expression is the Wnt/β-catenin pathway. Changes in β-catenin signalling throughout the day guide the circadian activation of PPAR. PPAR-gamma agonists inhibit β-catenin, whilst inhibition of β-catenin activates PPAR-gamma. This inverse relationship has significant implications for bone development. [22] Musculoskeletal complaints are frequent among patients treated with Accutane, with as many as half of patients reporting back pain. [23] This pain may reflect a potential reduction in bone mineral density and an increased risk of fracture, although it is highly dependent on dosing. [24] Many of Accutane's effects throughout the body, including those in bones, can be understood through its suppression of β-catenin.

It's therefore insightful to explain how this implicates PPAR through its relationship with β-catenin. Both osteoblasts (the cells that generate new bone) and adipocytes (fat cells) differentiate from the same common pluripotent precursor, mesenchymal stem cells. When PPAR-gamma is activated, it induces the growth of new adipocyte cells, whilst inhibiting the production of osteoblasts. [25] This is why activating the β-catenin pathway enhances bone growth, through suppressing PPAR-gamma mRNA expression. It could also be inferred that β-catenin signalling would therefore reduce adipogenesis. Suppressing PPAR-gamma can even enhance bone mass density, in a manner directly opposite to the effect of isotretinoin. [26]

The evidence from Accutane's effect on bones could be better understood as an increase in PPAR-gamma signalling with a concomitant reduction in β-catenin. This suggests that Accutane doesn't simply reduce PPAR-gamma signalling, and the exact direction of effect could vary between tissues. This prompts a re-evaluation of the evidence for the relationship between PPAR and Accutane. One of the markers for PPAR-gamma activity is adiponectin, a protein hormone secreted by adipocytes to regulate metabolism. Higher levels of adiponectin indicate increased PPAR-gamma expression. [27] Several studies have found that serum adiponectin is elevated after isotretinoin treatment. [28][29] The researchers even identified this as being paradoxical to the disturbances in serum lipids and glucose.

Given there's some evidence of Accutane directly increasing PPAR-gamma expression, [30] the metabolic disturbances of Accutane could be better understood through a mechanism implicating PPAR-alpha. The PPAR-alpha agonist Fenofibrate has the direct opposite effect to isotretinoin on free fatty acids and total cholesterol when administered to different experimental groups. [31] The role of PPAR-alpha might have been overlooked so far due to its relatively poor understanding when compared to PPAR-gamma. Based on the totality of evidence presented so far, it could be reasonable to conclude that PPAR-gamma is enhanced in some tissues in response to Accutane, whilst PPAR-alpha is repressed.

8.4 PPAR in The Brain: Dopamine and Endocannabinoids

It's clear that suppressing PPAR signalling can have adverse effects on metabolic health, but this may not be the most troubling consequence. It turns out that PPAR is highly expressed within certain regions of the brain. One of the regions where PPAR is highly expressed is in the midbrain dopaminergic neurons. Both PPAR-alpha and PPAR-gamma are found in 70% of these neurons, which play a pivotal role in the reward system.

Dopamine within the midbrain governs the response to rewarding stimuli, such as drugs, sex, and food. Furthermore, PPAR-alpha is expressed in 60% of glutamatergic neurons within the amygdala, and PPAR-gamma in 60% of GABAergic neurons. [18] One of the roles played by PPAR within these structures is the response to endocannabinoid signalling. Endocannabinoids such as anandamide exert a calming, anti-anxiety effect. Cannabinoids such as THC can activate PPAR-gamma, which is responsible for their neuroprotective effects in the treatment of Parkinson's disease. [19]

Researchers have found that PPAR-gamma in particular is required to facilitate the neurological effects of THC. They also identified that PPAR-alpha and PPAR-gamma can behave in distinct and opposing ways. For example, PPAR-gamma agonists reduce reward responses, and also THC-induced anxiety. Conversely, PPAR-alpha agonists enhance the response to rewarding stimuli.

Treatment with the PPAR-alpha agonist fenofibrate enhances dopaminergic response and motivation. The authors of the study characterize fenofibrate as possessing motivational and anti-anhedonic properties. [20] This starkly contrasts with the PPAR-gamma agonist pioglitazone, which is so effective at reducing reward response that it is a therapeutic option to treat substance abuse. [21] The opposite behaviour between PPAR-alpha and PPAR-gamma reflects the fact that they are inversely regulated. Heightened PPAR-gamma occurs with low PPAR-alpha signalling and vice versa.

8.5 Microbiome: Impact on hormones and neurosteroids

It's clear that PPARs can directly impact neurological function within the midbrain; however, there are other less direct ways by which PPARs are relevant to the brain. Palmitoylethanolamide (PEA) is an endogenous ligand for PPAR-alpha that stimulates the biosynthesis of allopregnanolone. [32] Allopregnanolone is a neurosteroid that acts as a natural sedative by functioning as a positive allosteric modulator of the GABA-A receptor. Artificial formulations of allopregnanolone have been found to be effective in treating postpartum depression and even PTSD. [33]

In healthy individuals, PEA increases in response to stress tests to activate PPAR-alpha, leading to a reduction in depressive or anxious symptoms. This has been found to be a consequence of increased allopregnanolone synthesis, stimulated by the increase in PEA binding to PPAR-alpha. [34] Poignantly, PEA levels have been observed to be lower in individuals suffering from PTSD. The interdependence between PPAR-alpha and allopregnanolone is highlighted by the fact that the usual pain relief provided by PEA was blocked by co-administration of finasteride, which inhibits allopregnanolone synthesis. [35]

PPAR-alpha and allopregnanolone also regulate emotional behaviour through the gut microbiome. It's well established that the gut is central to neurological health through the synthesis of neurosteroids and neurotransmitters, as well as short-chain fatty acids. Mood disorders are linked to gut health and inflammatory processes largely through PPAR-alpha activity. Both PPAR-alpha and allopregnanolone are highly expressed in the colon, where they have anti-inflammatory effects. [36] Additionally, PPAR-alpha influences the composition of the gut microbiome.

It's now evident that allopregnanolone and its relation to PPAR are key to understanding a variety of mood disorders, potentially including those linked to Accutane treatment. Allopregnanolone is synthesised through enzymes such as 3-alpha-HSD and 5-alpha reductase (5AR). In women with PTSD, it's been found that the low levels of allopregnanolone found in the cerebrospinal fluid are a consequence of impaired 3-alpha-HSD function. [37] In males suffering from the same condition, 5AR1 function was found to be at fault. [38] Intriguingly, Accutane has been found to have antiandrogenic properties by competitively inhibiting the action of 3-alpha-HSD, resulting in lower dihydrotestosterone (DHT) production. [39]

$$\text{Progesterone} \xrightarrow{5\alpha\text{-reductase}} 5\alpha\text{-Dihydroprogesterone} \xrightarrow{3\alpha\text{-HSD}} \text{Allopregnanolone}$$

It's likely that allopregnanolone is also therefore subjected to the same reduction. This effect would be further compounded by the almost threefold reduction in 5AR1 gene expression observed in skin biopsies after eight weeks of treatment with Accutane. [40] The change in 5AR1 expression could be attributed to changes in PPAR signalling, as PPAR ligands such as linoleic acid appear to have a synergistic effect on DHT synthesis. [41] Equally, blocking 5AR1 also lowers sebaceous lipid levels. The connection between PPAR-gamma and DHT works both ways, as DHT in turn induces PPAR-gamma expression. [42] A combination of both DHT and a PPAR-gamma activator dramatically increases sebocyte differentiation compared to a PPAR agonist or DHT alone. [43]

Androgen pathways aren't the only hormones influenced by Accutane. A novel PPAR-gamma agonist, MEKT1, was found to exert similar effects to Accutane in suppressing POMC (proopiomelanocortin) and ACTH (adrenocorticotropic hormone) secretion. [44] Isotretinoin is so effective in suppressing ACTH that it has been suggested as a treatment for Cushing's disease. [45] Accutane affects pituitary hormones through its regulation of the PPAR-gamma/RXR system. POMC is the prohormone to both ACTH and MSH (melanocyte-stimulating hormone). One intriguing property of melanocortins is facilitating sexual arousal. Artificial melanocortins have been proven to be effective in stimulating erections in men, and sexual desire. [46] PPAR-gamma activators induce cell-cycle arrest and apoptosis in ACTH-secreting pituitary tumours, favouring the notion that Accutane enhances PPAR-gamma activity to exert similar pituitary effects. [47]

8.6 Epigenetic Regulation of PPARs

As previously outlined, PPAR-alpha downregulation is implicated in mood disorders such as PTSD. Stress can influence epigenetics, and in a model of social isolation, it was found that PPAR-alpha can become hypermethylated in the hippocampi of rats. This leads to a deficiency in neurosteroid biosynthesis, as previously outlined. This effect was linked to an increase in histone deacetylase 1 (HDAC1) and methyl-CpG-binding protein 2 (MeCP2). The rats subjected to this social isolation became aggressive as a result of lower levels of allopregnanolone, highlighting the significance of epigenetic mechanisms in regulating PPAR signalling. [48]

Before going into the details of the epigenetic impact of PPAR signalling, it's important to give a brief introduction on what exactly epigenetics are. Epigenetics is the field of genetics that explains how gene expression can be altered without changing the underlying genetic code directly. Epigenetic mechanisms can essentially switch genes on and off in a lasting manner, and thereby influence an organism's traits and behaviour. Two twins sharing the same genes can experience vastly different health outcomes based on their exposure to epigenetic agents. There are two primary forms of epigenetic modification: DNA Methylation and Histone Modification.

Epigenetic modifications refer to alterations in how genes can be transcribed to take effect in the body. An analogy I've come up with to help make this easy to understand is to consider your genome as being like a book. Individual pages in the book could be thought of as genes. When a gene is transcribed, it's like reading from a particular page and copying it out by hand. An example of an epigenetic modification is DNA methylation, which makes the gene less accessible to transcriptional machinery. In this analogy methylation marks are like sticky tabs covering words in the page making it difficult (or impossible) to copy out the page - and so the gene can't be transcribed and translated into protein. So, the gene is said be to less 'expressed'.

Chromatin is a complex of DNA and protein that makes the DNA more compact, helping to regulate gene expression. When

Chromatin is tightly bundled it's less accessible to transcriptional machinery less gene transcription takes place. In this state it is referred to as heterochromatin. The oppose case is where it's more open and available for gene transcription where it's referred to as Euchromatin. When the chromatin is open and relaxed, or tightly closed, depends on Histone modifications. Acetyl groups can attach themselves to histone tails to encourage an open chromatin structure and therefore enhance gene transcription. However, these acetyl groups can also be removed by an enzyme call HDAC (Histone Deacetylase). Substances that can inhibit HDAC are referred to as HDACi's (Histone Deacetylase inhibitors) and can help relieve the lasting repression of particular genes.

PPAR signalling can both trigger HDAC inhibition, and HDAC inhibition can in turn enhance PPAR signalling. HDAC3 interacts with PPAR-gamma to deacetylate the protein, making it less available. Inhibiting HDAC3 can increase PPAR-gamma acetylation and enhance expression of target genes such as adiponectin. [49] Inhibiting HDAC3 is even sufficient to induce PPAR-gamma expression without the presence of a ligand. Butyrate is a naturally occurring short-chain fatty acid which is produced by fermentation of carbohydrates in the colon. It's also a potent epigenetic agent by acting as an HDAC inhibitor. Butyrate-forming bacteria play a role in connecting inflammatory bowel conditions, such as ulcerative colitis, to the body's epigenetic status. PPAR-alpha and PPAR-gamma have both been confirmed to be increased in response to butyrate supplementation. [50]

That pivotal connection between the microbiome and PPAR activity runs both ways, as PPAR-alpha activation can in turn improve microbiome composition. [51] PPAR activation reverses the downregulation of PPAR-alpha in rodent models of depression and anxiety, and in turn restores normal allopregnanolone levels. Berberine is a potent agonist of PPAR-alpha, and as such it corrects dysbiosis. In particular, the intestinal content of butyrate-forming bacteria is restored by metformin and berberine, relieving intestinal inflammation and ultimately repairing the intestinal barrier. [52]

8.7 Conclusion

The evidence shows that while the interaction between Accutane and PPAR is complex, it is also crucial to understanding both its efficacy in treating acne and its induction of side effects such as changes to blood lipids, bone density, and potentially even neurological effects. While PPAR agonists (both PPAR-gamma and PPAR-alpha) increase sebum production, the evidence that Accutane suppresses PPAR activity is mixed. It has been found that Accutane reduces PPAR-gamma expression in the Meibomian gland; however, one of the key markers for PPAR-gamma signalling, adiponectin, is found to be increased during treatment. The evidence also suggests that the metabolic disturbances linked to treatment with the acne drug might be better understood in terms of PPAR-alpha signalling.

While less well known than PPAR-gamma, PPAR-alpha is just as significant to metabolic health. In fact, studies have found that PPAR-alpha agonists are even more effective at inducing sebum production. The evidence for Accutane repressing PPAR-alpha signalling is supported by numerous studies showing that the retinoid inhibits β-catenin, a key signalling protein for cell proliferation linked to PPAR-alpha. Understanding Accutane's effects through a repression of PPAR-alpha signalling sheds light on the various side effects linked to the treatment, from gastrointestinal to psychological. It also presents a potential new approach in reversing these effects through supplementation with PPAR-alpha agonists such as PEA (Palmitoylethanolamide) or Berberine.

8.8 Chapter Summary

- **Complex Relationship Between Accutane and PPAR Signalling:** Accutane's effect on peroxisome proliferator-activated receptors (PPARs) is complex and sometimes contradictory. However, PPAR agonists like fibrates enhance sebum production whilst there's evidence Accutane suppresses PPAR signalling, impacting metabolic.

- **Mixed Effects on Insulin Sensitivity and Dyslipidaemia:** Accutane-induced dyslipidaemia should lead to decreased insulin sensitivity and higher circulating insulin levels, which seems counterintuitive for an acne treatment since insulin insensitivity is a known acne trigger. However, the evidence for Accutane impacting insulin is mixed.

- **Impact on PPAR-gamma and Meibomian Gland Dysfunction:** Accutane's suppression of PPAR-gamma is linked to Meibomian Gland Dysfunction (MGD), leading to dry eyes by reducing lipid secretion in these specialized sebaceous glands.

- **PPAR-gamma's Role in Retinoic Acid Signalling and Feedback Mechanism:** PPAR-gamma facilitates retinoic acid signalling by regulating enzymes like RDH10 and RALDH2 involved in its production.

- **Inverse Relationship Between β-catenin and PPAR-gamma:** The Wnt/β-catenin pathway regulates PPAR expression, where inhibition of β-catenin activates PPAR-gamma, and PPAR-gamma agonists inhibit β-catenin.

- **Accutane's Effects on Bone and β-catenin:** Accutane suppresses β-catenin signalling, which may lead to increased PPAR-gamma activity in some tissues. This may have an association with the joint and muscle pain experienced by some Accutane patients.

- **Variable Impact on PPAR-gamma and Metabolic Disturbances:** Evidence suggests that Accutane doesn't uniformly reduce PPAR-gamma signalling; instead, it may enhance PPAR-gamma expression in certain tissues. This is indicated by elevated serum adiponectin levels after treatment, which correlates with increased PPAR-gamma activity and may explain paradoxical disturbances in serum lipids and glucose.

- **Repression of PPAR-alpha and Metabolic Implications:** Accutane may repress PPAR-alpha, contributing to metabolic disturbances. PPAR-alpha agonists like fenofibrate have effects opposite to Accutane on free fatty acids and total cholesterol. This suggests that the metabolic side effects of Accutane could be better understood by considering its differential impact on PPAR-alpha and PPAR-gamma.

- **PPARs in Reward-Related Brain Regions:** PPAR-alpha and PPAR-gamma are highly expressed in key brain areas involved in the reward system, found in 70% midbrain dopaminergic neurons.

- **Role in Endocannabinoid Signalling and Neuroprotection:** PPAR-gamma can be activated by cannabinoids such as THC, facilitating their neuroprotective effects, especially in treating Parkinson's disease. Endocannabinoids like anandamide exert calming, anti-anxiety effects through PPARs.

- **Distinct and Opposing Effects of PPAR-alpha and PPAR-gamma Agonists:** PPAR-alpha and PPAR-gamma have opposite impacts on reward responses. PPAR-alpha agonists (e.g., fenofibrate) enhance dopaminergic response and motivation, possessing motivational and anti-anhedonic properties. In contrast, PPAR-gamma agonists (e.g., pioglitazone) reduce reward responses and THC-induced anxiety, making them useful in treating substance abuse.

- **Inverse Regulation of PPAR-alpha and PPAR-gamma:** The opposing behaviours of PPAR-alpha and PPAR-gamma reflect their inverse regulation—when PPAR-gamma levels are heightened, PPAR-alpha signalling is low, and vice versa—affecting reward processing and motivation.

- **PPAR-alpha Activation Increases Allopregnanolone Synthesis:** Palmitoylethanolamide (PEA), an endogenous ligand for PPAR-alpha, stimulates the production of allopregnanolone—a neurosteroid that acts as a natural sedative by modulating GABA-A receptors. This pathway reduces depressive and anxious symptoms and is significant in mood disorders like PTSD; Accutane may impact this pathway.

- **Regulation of Emotional Behaviour Through the Gut Microbiome:** PPAR-alpha and allopregnanolone influence emotional behaviour via the gut microbiome. They are highly expressed in the colon, where they have anti-inflammatory effects. Mood disorders are linked to gut health and inflammatory processes mediated largely by PPAR-alpha activity.

- **Accutane Inhibits Enzymes Critical for Neurosteroid and Hormone Synthesis:** Accutane inhibits 3-alpha-HSD and reduces 5AR1 gene expression—enzymes essential for synthesizing allopregnanolone and dihydrotestosterone (DHT). This leads to decreased levels of these neurosteroids and hormones, potentially contributing to mood disorders associated with Accutane treatment.

- **Impact on Pituitary Hormones via PPAR-gamma Activation:** Accutane affects pituitary hormones by enhancing PPAR-gamma activity, suppressing the secretion of POMC and ACTH, similar to the effects of PPAR-gamma agonists. This influences hormones like melanocortins, which facilitate sexual arousal, and may induce cell-cycle arrest and apoptosis in ACTH-secreting pituitary tumours.

9. Conclusion

9.1 Accutane's Extensive Effects

This book has presented the extensive and multifaceted adverse effects of Accutane (isotretinoin) treatment, in particular its significant impact on stem cell dynamics, retinoid metabolism, neurotransmitter systems, and overall neurological function.

Accutane converts into all-trans retinoic acid (ATRA), which modulates gene transcription through nuclear receptors like RAR and RXR. This modulation affects stem cell proliferation and differentiation by enhancing the degradation of β-catenin in the Wnt signalling pathway. While this mechanism is effective in treating severe acne by reducing uncontrolled cell growth, it may adversely affect tissues that rely on regular cell renewal—such as the skin, bones, gut, and brain—by depleting healthy stem cell populations and potentially leading to issues like decreased bone density and impaired intestinal function.

The drug disrupts the body's delicate retinoid metabolism, particularly involving enzymes that synthesize, store, and degrade retinoic acid. In particular there's evidence that enzymes in the ALDH family undergo lasting repression perhaps as some form of negative feedback. As a result, there is a decrease in endogenous synthesis of retinoic acid, as well as the many of the products of these enzymes outside of retinoic acid pathway, such as in metabolising the toxic products of dopamine transmission.

Accutane's influence extends to neurotransmitter systems, notably affecting dopamine and serotonin pathways. It may alter dopamine receptor gene transcription, potentially decreasing dopamine transmission and contributing to depressive symptoms and reduced motivation. Similarly, by increasing the levels of 5-HT1A autoreceptors in the Raphe Nuclei, Accutane can reduce serotonin availability in brain regions responsible for emotion, learning, and sexual behaviour, which might explain some mood alterations reported by patients.

Furthermore, Accutane appears to disrupt cognitive function by altering the balance between excitatory and inhibitory signals in the brain. Studies have observed decreased activity in the orbitofrontal cortex and changes in neurotransmitter receptor expression, leading to impairments in learning, memory, and mood regulation. The drug's effect on GABAergic and glutamatergic systems may contribute to significant neuropsychiatric side effects.

Given that the fundamental means by which Retinoic Acid exerts its broad effects throughout the body and brain is by opposing the Wnt/ β-catenin pathway, several chemicals become relevant in considering how these effects may be reversed. Specifically, Lithium, Melatonin and Butyrate all possess the ability to enhance β-catenin signalling and thereby encourage cell proliferation among other things. The most potent of these being Lithium. Lithium inhibits one of the components of the destruction complex, GSK3-β. This has the effect of boosting β-catenin in the brain, and in particular within the hippocampus. The conducive effect of Lithium on cell proliferation is so profound it even produces measurable differences in grey matter volume in patients being treated for bipolar.

One of the clearest effects in vitro findings for Isotretinoin's neurological impacts is that on 5-HT1A receptor. By dramatically increasing 5-HT1A autoreceptor protein levels in Raphe Nuclei cell cultures, Isotretinoin could significantly hamper serotonin transmission out into the rest of the brain. As it turns out, this finding could also possibly be explained by Isotretinoin's interaction with β-catenin as one of the main transcription factors for 5-HT1A expression, Deaf1, is regulated by GSK3-β. Since GSK3-β inactivates Deaf1, this could explain the increase 5-HT1A autoreceptor protein. This is why Lithium appears to enhance 5-HT1A expression at postsynaptic sites in the hippocampus, which could contribute to its antidepressant mechanism.

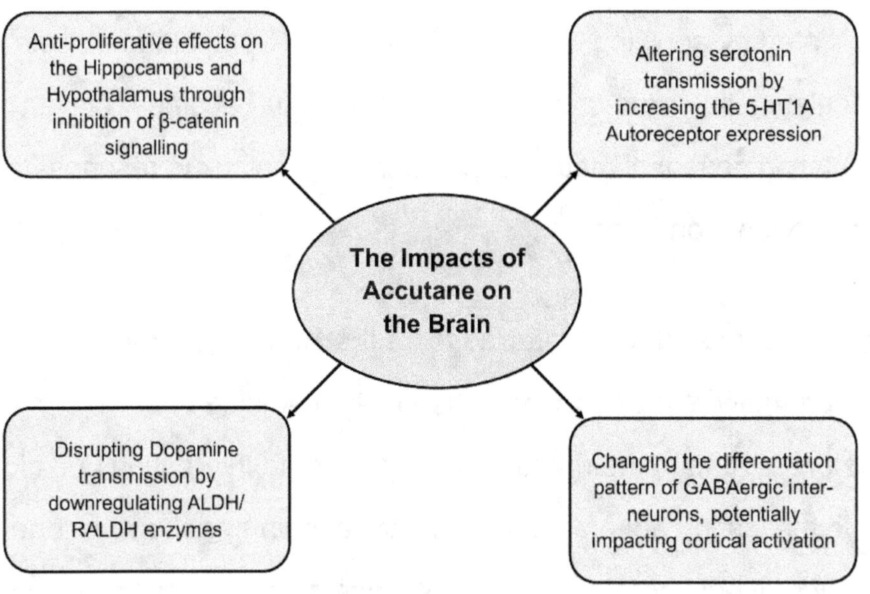

[Fig 14] The variety of documented effects of Retinoic Acid/Accutane on the brain.

Like Lithium, melatonin induces β-catenin signalling and enhances neurogenesis in both the hippocampus and hypothalamus. Melatonin's effects on cell proliferation even extend to dermal papilla cells, making it a promising, if unconventional, candidate for in vitro hair loss treatments. The interaction between melatonin and retinoic acid signalling is particularly intricate, as melatonin secretion and retinoic acid pathways in the brain appear to be co-regulated in response to photoreceptive changes over the diurnal cycle. Retinoic acid-regulated genes in the hypothalamus are inhibited during shorter photoperiods—an effect that can be replicated by applying melatonin. Given the hypothalamus's role in modulating sex hormone secretion, melatonin becomes relevant for regulating seasonal mating behaviours in livestock in response to varying light conditions.

This intricate system is referred to as the Retinohypothalamic axis, and primarily relies on the variation in light striking the photoreceptors in the retina. This raises some interesting questions as to the lasting adverse effects of Isotretinoin treatment, as one of the side effects best testified for its longevity is a reduction in night vision, believed to be a consequence of lasting inhibition of 11-cis-retinol dehydrogenase (11cRDH), a vital constituent of retinal photoreceptors. These same photoreceptors are also present in the brain, although the precise significance in the context of Isotretinoin is yet to be determined.

To explore ways of reversing the effects of Accutane, the focus should be on promoting processes that counteract its primary actions in the body — specifically, stem cell depletion and increased cellular turnover. These effects are largely driven by β-catenin inhibition through activation of the destruction complex. Throughout this book, several substances have been suggested for this purpose. The remainder of this chapter will examine how these compounds might be utilised to support tissue restoration in all organs affected by Accutane treatment.

9.2 Butyrate

Butyrate is a natural product of gut fermentation by the gut microbiota. As a short-chain fatty acid it has a number of vital roles in maintaining gut health, but also exerts some intriguing effects throughout the body. By enhancing β-catenin it can also help induce stem cell renewal in the intestinal epithelium. In fact, the ablation of β-catenin by Isotretinoin could itself contribute to the emergence of Inflammatory Bowel Diseases following treatment with the acne drug. Furthermore, Butyrate possesses some potent epigenetic effects by inhibiting HDAC and consequently enhancing gene transcription by encouraging a more open chromatin structure. The capacity for Butyrate to support renewal of stem cells may be particularly important in considering how some of the effects of Isotretinoin may be reversed.

Supplementation and Dosing

The way Butyrate regulates stem cell proliferation is fairly complex, and for the longest time left researchers perplexed. Whilst low doses of Butyrate appear to encourage cell proliferation in vivo, high doses appear to do the opposite. This apparent contradiction has been called the 'Butyrate Paradox'. This is why that Butyrate has been found to be beneficial to treating colorectal cancer, which wouldn't be expected from a chemical that only encouraged tissue growth and proliferation. [1] Nonetheless, the evidence for Butyrate for protecting against apoptosis is extensive, through promoting the release of a variety of stimulatory growth factors such as insulin-like growth factor-2 (IGF-2). [2] The consensus among scientists is that under normal healthy conditions, the beneficial effects of Butyrate on cell proliferation of epithelial cells predominates. This is why direct administration of Butyrate via enema can even speed up tissue repair following intestinal surgery. [3]

The most effective substrate for encouraging the activity of Butyrate is resistant starch when it escapes digestion. These starches are then fermented by butyrate producing bacteria such as Ruminococcaceae. Increasing dietary sources of Butyrate can significantly elevate both Butyrate concentrations, and Butyrate producing bacteria. For example, one study of 174 university students found that supplementing certain dietary starches could dramatically increase short-chain fatty acid (SCFA) production, as well as increase the relative abundance of butyrate-producing bacteria. [5] These bacteria in the colon are able to break down the complex polysaccharides in these starches that we simply don't have the enzymes to break down ourselves.

The starch that was most effective at increasing SCFA production was that from potatoes, giving an increase in SCFA concentrations of 32% after just two weeks. Supplementing Inulin was also effective with a 12% increase in SCFA concentrations. Potato starches were especially effective at raising Butyrate concentrations with a 29% elevation, which was associated with increases in **Ruminococcus bromii** or **Clostridium chartatabidum**. The researchers note that Potato Starch is specifically effective at stimulating Butyrate production over Inulin or Maize starches, and this wasn't dependent on dosing either with similar results being achieved with doses ranging from 24g to 34g of resistant potato starch. Cooking potatoes reduces the quantity of resistant starch from 4.27g/100g to 3.00g/100g. [6] This means in order to obtain 30 grams of resistant potato starch without supplementation, it would require ingesting around 1kg of potatoes, which is impractical.

Direct supplementation of Butyrate not only exerts beneficial effects on gut health, but also **metabolic health** and **inflammation**. One animal study investigated the effects of Butyrate on modifying the response to **exercise** and **lipid metabolism** in mice fed a high fat diet. Supplementing Butyrate significantly reversed the metabolic damage caused by the high fat diet. [7] Interestingly, **exercise**

alone was also able to enhance Butyrate-producing bacteria in faecal samples.

Over the 8-week study period, the high fat cohort experienced a dramatic increase in body weight, with a diet consisting of 45% of calories coming from fat. Administering Butyrate along with the high fat diet prevented this increase in weight gain. Butyrate also decreased the amount of white adipose tissue in the gonadal and liver samples. Butyrate supplementation also partially remediated the increase in pro-inflammatory cytokines such as TNF-α and IL-1β caused by the high fat diet. The dose of Sodium Butyrate used in this study was 300 mg/kg/day, which equates to around 1.7 g total for the average adult. However, some questions remain as to the effect of chronic Butyrate supplementation on gut flora composition, with evidence that it may increase the abundance of Firmicutes at the expense of Bacteroidetes. [8]

Interactions with PPARs

Aside from its effects on the gut, Butyrate has another property that make it especially relevant to reversing the effects of Accutane treatment. Treatment with the acne drug has been linked to a number of metabolic disturbances, perhaps mediated through the PPAR receptors (Peroxisome Proliferator-Activated Receptors). As well as being involved in metabolic processes such as lipid metabolism and glucose regulation, PPARs are directly implicated in sebum production. As previously discussed, sebum is the oily substance secreted from sebaceous glands throughout the body, including the very important glands that sit around the rim of the eyes. These specialised sebum glands are called the meibomian glands, and the oily secretions they produce protect the surface layer of the eye.

One of the many complaints of Accutane treatment is a persistent dry eyes, called Meibomian Gland Dysfunction. Investigations into the cause of this effect have found that Accutane significantly impairs PPAR-gamma activity in the meibomian gland, and thereby hampering lipid production. [9] Butyrate supplementation can positively modulate PPAR-gamma to not only yield beneficial effects for insulin sensitivity and adipogenesis, but perhaps therefore also sebum production too. [10] In fact, another PPAR agonist, Berberine, has even been found to be effective in protecting sebocytes from cell death and improving tear film production. This is why Berberine has even been included as an ingredient in eye drops by companies like Murine.

9.3 ALCAR (Acetyl-L-carnitine)

Acetyl-L-carnitine (ALCAR) is a naturally occurring compound derived from L-carnitine that supports energy metabolism in the body. Unlike L-carnitine, ALCAR can easily cross the blood-brain barrier, where it has unique benefits, particularly relevant in the context of Accutane treatment. ALCAR has been shown to upregulate the enzyme ALDH1A1, which plays a vital role in detoxification processes. [11] Many of the adverse effects of Accutane treatment can be linked to a lasting repression of these detoxifying enzymes, including the lasting repression of night vision as well as perhaps changes in the dopaminergic system.

Supplementation and Dosing

One proposed mechanism for ALCAR's effect involves its enhancement of β-catenin signalling, a recurring topic in this text. By inhibiting GSK3-β, ALCAR is able to boost β-catenin which I've presented evidence to suggest plays a key role in regulating ALDH activity through a hypothetical negative feedback loop. Strengthening ALDH activity in the brain allows ALCAR to break down neurotoxic byproducts of dopamine metabolism, like DOPAL, which helps elevate synaptic dopamine levels while protecting neurons from toxicity and cell death. The dosage in this study was relatively high compared to common over-the-counter supplements, amounting to roughly 1.2g for a 70 kg individual.

Androgen Receptor

Carnitine's benefits aren't just limited to upregulating ALDH activity, but also in enhancing androgen signalling via the androgen receptor. Research has demonstrated a profound impact of isotretinoin on the androgen receptor (AR). A specific study observed a significant decrease in AR-positive cells in male skin biopsies after a 12-week isotretinoin treatment, dropping from 26.6% to 20.6%.[60] Furthermore, the researchers identified a minor yet statistically insignificant alteration in AR binding affinity (from 0.44 to 0.32 nmol/L), coupled with a more substantial 2.6-fold reduction in binding capacity.[61] Binding capacity, in this context, refers to the concentration of receptors in the cytosol.

β-Catenin plays a critical role as a co-regulator of the androgen receptor (AR). Its cytoplasmic levels increase in response to Wnt signalling, which inhibits GSK3 activity within the destruction complex. In this capacity, β-catenin binds to the ligand-binding domain (LBD) of the AR, thereby modulating the transcriptional functions of the AR's N-terminal domain (NTD). The N-terminal domain provides a binding platform for approximately 150 co-regulators and co-repressors, which finely tune the AR's activity upon activation by androgens such as dihydrotestosterone (DHT). [62]

Researchers have discovered that it may be possible to increase androgen receptor sensitivity by supplementing carnitine. A study of 10 resistance-trained men were supplemented with L-carnitine in the form L-carnitine L-tartrate (LCLT) for 3 weeks before taking muscle biopsies. [63] The researchers were aiming to investigate how supplementing L-carnitine may modulate the response to exercise in the short period after training has been completed.

It's known that the androgen receptor is influenced by training alone, since AR mRNA (although not protein) is elevated 48 hours after training. [64] However there is a relevant lack of research on the impact of resistance training on androgen receptors immediately after training. It's been hypothesised that L-carnitine supplementation could preserve androgen receptors in muscle tissue that been broken down during training, and thereby improve recovery.

The test group consumed a total of 2g of L-carnitine evenly split across breakfast and lunch each day. The morning training regimen consisted of a typical compound movement routine including bench press, squat, bent-over row, and shoulder press. The biopsies from the quadricep leg muscles revealed a dramatic increase in AR content versus control. Additionally, feeding after the training further enhanced AR content compared to pre-training values. The researchers also found that there was also a greater cellular uptake in testosterone as compared to control.

The impact of carnitine supplementation on androgen signalling is so profound that it's even been found analogous to testosterone replacement therapy. A study of 120 patients given either testosterone undecanoate, carnitine (2g of propionyl-l-carnitine per day with acetyl-l-carnitine 2g per day) or placebo, found that both testosterone and carnitine significantly improved erectile function and reduced fatigue. [65]

In fact, the carnitine protocol proved to be significantly more effective at improving nocturnal erections than testosterone. Acetyl-l-carnitine (ALCAR) might have an advantage in being better at crossing the blood brain barrier than other preparations. [66] I've previously highlighted the beneficial role of ALCAR is restoring ALDH activity, perhaps mediated through an increase in β-catenin signalling.

9.4 Melatonin

In a previous chapter, I outlined the substantial evidence linking retinoid signalling and melatonin in the brain. In many respects, melatonin and retinoic acid exert opposing effects in various brain structures, notably in the hypothalamus and pineal gland. One key difference lies in their impact on cell proliferation: melatonin promotes stem cell proliferation, whereas retinoic acid inhibits it, including in the hippocampus. [12] [13] In a 2004 study by Crandall et al., 42 days of treatment with retinoic acid almost halved the proliferation of hippocampal stem cells. [14] This finding corroborates the evidence from other studies that treatment with Isotretinoin can impact memory formation.

Supplementation and Dosing

The diverging effects between retinoic acid and melatonin include the impact on beta-catenin signalling, which is enhanced by melatonin and inhibited by retinoic acid. Furthermore, it appears that retinoic acid synthesis and melatonin secretion are alternatively regulated in the brain throughout the diurnal cycle. Direct injections of melatonin to the hypothalamus result in reductions in the activity of enzymes involved in synthesising retinoic acid such as Raldh1. [15]

Exogenous supplementation of melatonin can dramatically enhance hippocampal neurogenesis and cell proliferation by 90%, after 3, 6 and 9 months. [16] Interestingly the doses used in these animal studies can vary dramatically. [17] Melatonin at above 2.5 mg/kg can significantly increase the number doublecortin-positive neurons as well as the number and complexity of dendrite trees. Similarly beneficial effects were observed in a study using 8mg/kg which assessed the effect on depressive like behaviour in a force swim test.

9.5 Lithium

Among all the supplements discussed in this book, lithium stands out as the one most directly opposing the broad spectrum of effects produced by retinoic acid in the body. This opposition is evident in lithium's potential to cause acne, highlighting its contrasting mechanism. Lithium's mode of action can be seen as the mirror opposite of retinoic acid, particularly due to its impact on cytoplasmic β-catenin levels, which it raises in a way fundamentally different from Accutane. Lithium functions as an agonist of the canonical Wnt signalling pathway by inhibiting GSK3-β activity, which, in turn, releases β-catenin from the destruction complex. Through this mechanism, lithium promotes cell proliferation throughout the body, including in the brain. Chronic high-dose lithium treatment in human hippocampal cultures has been shown to increase the production of progenitor cells, neuroblasts, and neurons. [18][19]

Supplementation and Dosing

When considering supplementing with Lithium, the most important factor to address is dosing. Lithium's bad reputation largely stems from the almost toxic doses used in treating depression and bipolar disorder, where doses of up to 900mg of lithium carbonate are administered multiple times a day. [20] This far exceeds the amount of lithium one could expect to absorb naturally through ground water, which may be as much as 0.5mg depending on your location. [21] At these much lower 'microdoses', the beneficial effects of lithium on brain health become much more apparent without the side effects associated with clinical dosing. [22]

The contrasting effects between high and low dose regimes gives rise to some apparent paradoxes. For example, lithium treatment for mania is often associated with hair loss, however studies have shown that low dose topical lithium actually improves hair growth. [23][24] As it turns out, the toxic clinical doses of lithium disrupts thyroid function, which has a knock-on effect on hair growth. The proliferative effect of lithium on dermal papilla cells (the cells that form hair) is much more in line with lithium's general mechanism of action.

At what dose of Lithium does the cost-to-benefit analysis begin to skew in the other direction? Well, what's surprising is just how little lithium is needed to have a measurably positive effect. A 15-month trial of a so-called lithium 'microdose' of just 0.3mg was found to all but halt the progression of Alzheimer's disease. In the final analysis, the group that was treated with the lithium microdose showed no decrease in performance in cognitive tests, in contrast to the control group which did experience cognitive decline. [25]

Other animal studies on 'microdoses' of lithium have found that just 0.25mg/Kg/day added to drinking water significantly improved spatial memory, as well as decreased amyloid plaque precursors. [26]

Slightly higher doses, which could be better considered as being in the low-therapeutic range, similarly show benefits. A trial of just 150mg of lithium carbonate has been found effective in treating ADHD and addiction disorders. [27] The results are striking for just how well the treatment was tolerated. The patients reported improvements in sleep, mood and general hopefulness, with one patient stating: "I feel like this really made a difference, I'm just…better." This low dose was all but absent of side effects, including sexual side effects typically manifest with other antidepressant treatments. 150mg of lithium carbonate translates to around 28mg of active lithium, which is still significantly greater than supplemental doses or what's available through ground water.

It's clear that both low-dose and microdoses of lithium treatments are all but free of side effects whilst maintaining efficacy. It would now be reasonable to question at what point lithium begins to manifest toxic effects or hormonal disturbances. One animal study investigated the impact of three different doses of lithium chloride on endocrine function at 0.1 mg, 0.2 mg and 0.4 mg/100 g body weight/day for 21 days. [28] At the end of the study the researchers measured the impact of the treatment on testicular enzymes and several sex hormones. Only the lowest dose of 0.1mg (per 100g body weight) had no effect on 3β -HSD and 17β -HSD, with no changes to testosterone and other sex hormones. The highest dose of 0.4 mg/100g showed the strongest detrimental effect on fertility parameters and hormones. It's clear that hormonal effects are highly dose dependent.

Meta-analysis have called into question the high doses typically used in treating bipolar and depression given the risk of toxicity, especially since benefits still manifest at 'sub-therapeutic' doses. [29] In fact, ionic lithium at 5mg or less, especially from dietary sources, has even been found to be kidney protective. [30] The research on low dose lithium remains scant, nonetheless it's reasonable to conclude that up to 5mg of ionic lithium maintains a favourable balance between neurological benefits and health outcomes.

Boosting Lithium with B-vitamins

Another compelling advantage of lithium supplementation is its positive impact on B-vitamin metabolism, which may be especially beneficial in mitigating the side effects of Accutane treatment. Among Accutane's many side effects, one of the most significant is the elevation of homocysteine levels. Accutane appears to disrupt normal B12 and folate metabolism, leading to increased homocysteine levels in the blood. This occurs because folic acid and B12 act as cofactors in the recycling of homocysteine into methionine through a process called transmethylation. Methionine is an essential amino acid involved in several critical functions, including methylation and protein synthesis. Given methionine's fundamental role, its depletion—along with the resulting increase in homocysteine—can have widespread adverse effects on the body. Symptoms of elevated homocysteine, or Hyperhomocysteinemia, include cardiovascular damage, cerebrovascular diseases, atherosclerosis, and even depression. [31]

The exact mechanism by which Accutane suppresses B12 and folate is not fully understood, but it appears to partially involve the inhibition of the enzyme cystathionine-β-synthase, which is essential for homocysteine metabolism. [32] However, the potential consequences for patients are well-established and can be severe if left unaddressed. Given the importance of B12 and folate in neurotransmitter production, some researchers even attribute Accutane's psychiatric effects primarily to this suppression. [33] Interestingly the reduction in B12 might even constitute one of Accutane therapeutic pathways in the treatment of acne. B12 supplementation can actually exacerbate acne development by altering gene transcription of the microbiota on the surface of the skin. [34]

One of the organs in which symptoms of Hyperhomocysteinemia manifests is in the musculoskeletal system. Excessive homocysteine increases osteoclast (cells that break down bone) activity, and results in an increased risk for bone fracture and osteoporosis. There's even been six recorded case reports of Accutane patients suffering from musculoskeletal discomfort being treated with B12 and folate, and then recovering from their symptoms. [35] These patients received shots of B12 every two weeks with 1mg of Folic acid daily and after 6 weeks of treatment symptoms "completely disappeared", although the treatment was continued for another five months. I've highlighted the significance of β-catenin in explaining the many diverse and lasting symptoms of Accutane treatment, including skeletal aberrations. Incredibly it appears that B12 is able to support the canonical Wnt/β-catenin pathway by acting as a Wnt surrogate. [36][37]

Folic acid has repeatedly been identified as a tool in offsetting the psychiatric effects of Isotretinoin, on account of its normalising effect on homocysteine and neurotransmitters. [38] However there's been increasing evidence that folate instead mediates its anti-depressant effect through GSK3-beta inhibition. [39] In a forced-to-swim test in mice, the treatment of a PI3K inhibitor or PPAR-gamma antagonist prevented the antidepressant effect on folic acid supplementation.

Additionally, folic acid has been shown to significantly enhance the antidepressant effect of lithium. This may help explain findings from the mid-1980s, which demonstrated that folic acid supplementation notably improved lithium's efficacy in treating patients with bipolar disorder and depression. [40] The mutual potentiation of Lithium and B12/folate can be further demonstrated with the evidence that Lithium may also improve the cellular absorption of B12. [41] Researchers found a positive correlation between lithium supplementation and the B12 marker cobalt in hair samples, reinforcing in vitro studies that suggest lithium improves cellular uptake of B12.

One of the more common complaints by those undergoing clinical dosing of Lithium is a feeling of reduced energy and general somnolence. For those being treated for mania, a bit less energy might actually be beneficial – but in treating PAS it makes higher doses undesirable. It isn't exactly known how Lithium causes this effect, but the leading theory is that it reduces the concentration of a particular sugar called Inositol (also known as vitamin B8) in some regions of the brain. [42] By depleting inositol in some regions of the brain, Lithium can attenuate intracellular signalling. [43]

People on average already ingest around 1g of inositol through their diet, but there's some encouraging evidence that supplementing 6g of inositol daily can offset dermatological side effects caused by clinical Lithium dosing. [44] Furthermore, a tailored protocol using an 80:1 ratio of myo-inositol and d-chiro-inositol totalling 4 grams proved to be effective in mitigating a spectrum of peripheral Lithium effects, including thyroid, cardiac and weight parameters. [45] This study found that supplementing in this way can dramatically improve the tolerability of those undergoing Lithium treatment for depression or mania.

9.6 PPARs

Of all the pathways influenced by Accutane treatment, PPAR receptors appear to be the most fundamental to its therapeutic effect in treating acne. Other than androgens, PPAR receptors are the only pathway known to influence sebum production – and in fact, it's believed that androgens induce sebum primarily via the PPAR receptors. PPARs directly regulate lipid metabolism, cell proliferation and differentiation – all processes that are heavily implicated in both the desired effect of Accutane treatment as well as the unintended side effects too. Unfortunately, these receptors are still somewhat mysterious despite being highly coveted by pharmaceutical companies wanting to develop diet pills. [46] However, the unpredictability of medications targeting these receptors has meant that as of yet, their use is still limited.

Medications that bind to these receptors can induce sebum production, such as thiazolidinediones or fibrates. [47]

Meibomian Gland Dysfunction

A study comparing the relative effects of PPAR-alpha and PPAR-gamma agonists on sebum production found that patients treated with fibrates (PPAR-alpha agonist) induced a 77% increase in sebum production, whilst thiazolidinediones (PPAR-gamma) treatment gave a 37% increase. The clearest evidence for the impact of Isotretinoin on PPAR signalling comes from an animal study investigating the development of Meibomian Gland Dysfunction ('dry eyes'). They found that treatment with the acne drug reduced PPAR-γ expression, which likely explains the reduction in lipogenesis. [48] However, there's also reason to believe that Accutane treatment could disrupt PPAR-alpha activity too. [49]

PPAR receptors are responsible for androgen induction of lipogenesis, resulting in oily skin. When combined with the strongest natural androgen, dihydrotestosterone (DHT), PPAR-gamma agonists can potentiate the sebum induction. [50] When combining DHT with a PPAR-gamma agonist (BRL-49653), the number of differentiated lipid-producing cells increased from 25% to 80%. Androgens are the primary regulators of sebaceous gland activity, individuals who lack a functional androgen receptor do not produce sebum and are therefore unable to develop acne. [51]

Cross-talk with Androgens

As previously detailed, Accutane downregulates key enzymes involved in the endogenous synthesis of retinoic acid, such as Retinol Dehydrogenase enzymes. When Isotretinoin downregulates these Retinol Dehydrogenases, it not only disrupts retinoid signalling but also hormone cascades too. For example, the repression of Retinol Dehydrogenase-4 by Accutane inhibits the production of the very potent androgen dihydrotestosterone (DHT), which might contribute to its anti-acne effects. [52] Due to the cross-talk between PPAR signalling and androgens, reduced sebum production and the consequent meibomian gland dysfunction is often observed in individuals with androgen insensitivity syndrome. [53]

This association has prompted researchers to attempt to remediate the meibomian gland dysfunction caused by Accutane with the administration of DHEA (dehydroepiandrosterone), an androgen precursor. They found that Accutane treatment of 0.5 mg/kg/day for 3 months dramatically reduced the activity of the androgen receptor in acinar cells in the ducts of the meibomian glands. [54] However, twice daily administration of a 1% DHEA solution to the eyes remediated this effect, and effectively restored normal Meibomian gland function.

This finding parallels observations from a study on women with Sjögren's syndrome, an autoimmune condition with notable similarities to many side effects associated with Accutane treatment. Sjögren's syndrome is marked by the destruction of exocrine glands, including sebaceous glands, tear ducts, and salivary glands. One of its primary symptoms is excessively dry skin, drawing a strong comparison to the dryness often experienced with Accutane use. Additional symptoms—such as dry eyes, fatigue, and muscle and joint pain—are also commonly reported by individuals undergoing Accutane treatment.

The "dryness" characteristic of Sjögren's syndrome affects various mucosal tissues, extending to the airways, digestive tract, and reproductive organs. As previously stated, exocrine glands are highly responsive to sex hormones. One particular cell type that's used to illustrate the androgens are acinar cells. These acinar glands are protected by the potent male androgen Dihydrotestosterone (DHT) and are better protected against atrophy and cell death (apoptosis) in men. In women it's believed that the failure to locally synthesise DHT from the hormone precursor DHEA is a significant contributor to the loss of epithelial cell renewal in Sjogren's syndrome. [55]

PPAR Agonists

A natural PPAR agonist is Berberine, which is an alkaloid of plants such as barberry. There is also evidence that Berberine mediates its effects through modulating PPAR, although the direction of this effect might vary between tissues. For example, Berberine increases PPAR-gamma expression in macrophages. [56] One striking discovery is that Berberine could even protect sebocytes (comparable to the cells in the meibomian gland) from apoptosis when coupled with another anti-diabetic agent, metformin. [57] A more direct application of berberine eye drops could improve tear production through modulating inflammation and PI3K pathways, making in effective in remediating dry eyes. There are even supplemental formulations of Berberine eyedrops specifically for this purpose.

An endogenous ligand of PPAR is Palmitoylethanolamide (PEA), which can bind to PPAR-alpha to exert beneficial effects on the brain and on reducing inflammation. Palmitoylethanolamide (PEA) can also stimulate the biosynthesis of Allopregnanolone. Allopregnanolone is a neurosteroid which is a natural sedative, by acting as positive allosteric modulator of the GABA-a receptor. Artificial formulations of Allopregnanolone has been found to be effective in treating postpartum depression and even PTSD. [58][59] In healthy individuals PEA increases in response to stress tests to activate PPAR-a, leading to a reduction in depressive or anxious symptoms. This has been found to be a consequence of increased allopregnanolone synthesis, stimulated by the increase in PEA binding to PPAR-alpha.

9.6 Reversing the Effects of Accutane

Combining all the interventions mentioned above would create a supplement stack capable of effectively counteracting the wide range of in vitro effects associated with Accutane and high-dose retinoic acid more broadly:

- **Butyrate: 500mg with 30 grams of resistant potato starch. Supplementing with Sodium Butyrate exerts rapid effects, whilst supplementing with resistant potato starch encourages longer term endogenous synthesis of Butyrate**
- **Acetyl-L-Carnitine: 1-2g. L-carnitine L-tartrate could be added given the evidence for its beneficial effect on androgen signalling via the androgen receptor. ALCAR can have an 'activating' effect, so it's encouraged to take in the morning so as not disrupt sleep.**
- **Melatonin: 1-5mg before bed.**

- **Lithium: 1-5mg**

- **B-complex: B-vitamins such as B12 and folate are shown to remediate the effect of elevated homocysteine levels that can be caused by Accutane treatment. There's direct evidence for this resolving the musculoskeletal pain that's caused by Hyperhomocysteinemia as result of Accutane. Additionally, Inositol can ameliorate some of the peripheral effects of Lithium, which can in turn enhance the absorption of B12.**

10. References

Chapter 1 References

[1] https://www.newsweek.com/accutane-murder-acne-drug-defense-821437

[2] Monica Cojoc, Claudia Peitzsch, Ina Kurth, Franziska Trautmann, Leoni A. Kunz-Schughart, Gennady D. Telegeev, Eduard A. Stakhovsky, John R. Walker, Karl Simin, Stephen Lyle, Susanne Fuessel, Kati Erdmann, Manfred P. Wirth, Mechthild Krause, Michael Baumann, Anna Dubrovska; Aldehyde Dehydrogenase Is Regulated by β-catenin/TCF and Promotes Radioresistance in Prostate Cancer Progenitor Cells. Cancer Res 1 April 2015; 75 (7): 1482–1494. https://doi.org/10.1158/0008-5472.CAN-14-1924

[3] Int J Environ Res Public Health. 2022 Jun; 19(11): 6463. Published online 2022 May 26. doi: 10.3390/ijerph19116463

[4] https://www.futuremarketinsights.com/reports/retinoids-market

[5] Rheinwald JG, Hahn WC, Ramsey MR, Wu JY, Guo Z, Tsao H, De Luca M, Catricalà C, O'Toole KM. A two-stage, p16(INK4A)- and p53-dependent keratinocyte senescence mechanism that limits replicative potential independent of telomere status. Mol Cell Biol. 2002 Jul;22(14):5157-72. doi: 10.1128/MCB.22.14.5157-5172.2002. PMID: 12077343; PMCID: PMC139780.

[6] Weinstein GD, Nigra TP, Pochi PE, Savin RC, Allan A, Benik K, Jeffes E, Lufrano L, Thorne EG. Topical tretinoin for treatment of photodamaged skin. A multicenter study. Arch Dermatol. 1991 May;127(5):659-65. PMID: 2024983.

[7] Fisher GJ, Datta SC, Talwar HS, Wang ZQ, Varani J, Kang S, Voorhees JJ. Molecular basis of sun-induced premature skin ageing and retinoid antagonism. Nature. 1996 Jan 25;379(6563):335-9. doi: 10.1038/379335a0. PMID: 8552187.

[8] Lee DD, Stojadinovic O, Krzyzanowska A, Vouthounis C, Blumenberg M, Tomic-Canic M. Retinoid-responsive transcriptional changes in epidermal keratinocytes. J Cell Physiol. 2009 Aug;220(2):427-439. doi: 10.1002/jcp.21784. PMID: 19388012; PMCID: PMC4386731.

[9] https://www.gov.uk/drug-safety-update/isotretinoin-roaccutane-rare-reports-of-erectile-dysfunction-and-decreased-libido

[10] https://content.iospress.com/articles/international-journal-of-risk-and-safety-in-medicine/jrs210023

Chapter 2 References

[1] Vitamin A and retinoid signaling: genomic and nongenomic effects Al Tanoury, Ziad et al. Journal of Lipid Research, Volume 54, Issue 7, 1761 – 1775

[2][3] Saari, J.C. (1999). Retinoids in Mammalian Vision. In: Nau, H., Blaner, W.S. (eds) Retinoids. Handbook of Experimental Pharmacology, vol 139. Springer, Berlin, Heidelberg. https://doi.org/10.1007/978-3-642-58483-1_20

[4] Retinoic Acid: Its Biosynthesis and Metabolism Joseph L. Napoli https://doi.org/10.1016/S0079-6603(08)60722-9

[5] Tsukada M, Schröder M, Roos TC, Chandraratna RA, Reichert U, Merk HF, Orfanos CE, Zouboulis CC. 13-cis retinoic acid exerts its specific activity on human sebocytes through selective intracellular isomerization to all-trans retinoic acid and binding to retinoid acid receptors. J Invest Dermatol. 2000 Aug;115(2):321-7. doi: 10.1046/j.1523-1747.2000.00066.x. PMID: 10951254.

[6] Olson JM, Ameer MA, Goyal A. Vitamin A Toxicity. [Updated 2023 Sep 2]. In: StatPearls [Internet]. Treasure Island (FL): StatPearls Publishing; 2024 Jan- . Available from: https://www.ncbi.nlm.nih.gov/books/NBK532916/

[7] Ina Strate, Tan H. Min, Dobromir Iliev, Edgar M. Pera; Retinol dehydrogenase 10 is a feedback regulator of retinoic acid signalling during axis formation and patterning of the central nervous system. Development 1 February 2009; 136 (3): 461–472. doi: https://doi.org/10.1242/dev.024901

[8] Generation of Retinaldehyde for Retinoic Acid Biosynthesis Biomolecules 2020, 10(1), 5; https://doi.org/10.3390/biom10010005

[9] Valenta T, Hausmann G, Basler K. The many faces and functions of β-catenin. EMBO J. 2012 Jun 13;31(12):2714-36. doi: 10.1038/emboj.2012.150. Epub 2012 May 22. PMID: 22617422; PMCID: PMC3380220.

[10] Zhu X, Wang W, Zhang X, Bai J, Chen G, Li L, Li M. All-Trans Retinoic Acid-Induced Deficiency of the Wnt/β-catenin Pathway Enhances Hepatic Carcinoma Stem Cell Differentiation. PLoS One. 2015 Nov 16;10(11):e0143255. doi: 10.1371/journal.pone.0143255. PMID: 26571119; PMCID: PMC4646487.

[11] On the role of Wnt/β-catenin signaling in stem cells Susanne J. Kühl, Michael Kühl Biochimica et Biophysica Acta (BBA) - General Subjects https://doi.org/10.1016/j.bbagen.2012.08.010

[12] All-trans-retinoic acid inhibits growth of head and neck cancer stem cells by suppression of Wnt/β-catenin pathway European Journal of Cancer Young Chang Lim [a], Hyun Jung Kang [a], Young Sook Kim [a], Eun Chang Choi https://doi.org/10.1016/j.ejca.2012.04.013

[13] Tsukada M, Schröder M, Roos TC, Chandraratna RA, Reichert U, Merk HF, Orfanos CE, Zouboulis CC. 13-cis retinoic acid exerts its specific activity on human sebocytes through selective intracellular isomerization to all-trans retinoic acid and binding to retinoid acid receptors. J Invest Dermatol. 2000 Aug;115(2):321-7. doi: 10.1046/j.1523-1747.2000.00066.x. PMID: 10951254.

[14] Gudas, L.J. and Wagner, J.A. (2011), Retinoids regulate stem cell differentiation. J. Cell. Physiol., 226: 322-330. https://doi.org/10.1002/jcp.22417

Chapter 3 References

[1] Olson JM, Ameer MA, Goyal A. Vitamin A Toxicity. [Updated 2023 Sep 2]. In: StatPearls [Internet]. Treasure Island (FL): StatPearls Publishing; 2024 Jan-. Available from: https://www.ncbi.nlm.nih.gov/books/NBK532916/

[2] Ina Strate, Tan H. Min, Dobromir Iliev, Edgar M. Pera; Retinol dehydrogenase 10 is a feedback regulator of retinoic acid signalling during axis formation and patterning of the central nervous system. Development 1 February 2009; 136 (3): 461–472. doi: https://doi.org/10.1242/dev.024901

[3] Belyaeva, O.V.; Adams, M.K.; Popov, K.M.; Kedishvili, N.Y. Generation of Retinaldehyde for Retinoic Acid Biosynthesis. Biomolecules 2020, 10, 5. https://doi.org/10.3390/biom10010005

[4] Lee, Haeok PhD, RN, FAAN; Kim, Sun S. PhD, RN; You, Kwang Soo PhD, RN; Park, Wanju PhD, RN, NPc; Yang, Jin Hyang PhD, RN; Kim, Minjin MSN, RN; Hayman, Laura L. PhD, RN, FAAN. Asian Flushing: Genetic and Sociocultural Factors of Alcoholism Among East Asians. Gastroenterology Nursing 37(5):p 327-336, September/October 2014. | DOI: 10.1097/SGA.0000000000000062

[5] Yu, RL., Tan, CH., Lu, YC. et al. Aldehyde dehydrogenase 2 is associated with cognitive functions in patients with Parkinson's disease. Sci Rep 6, 30424 (2016). https://doi.org/10.1038/srep30424

[6] Jonathan A. Doorn, Virginia R. Florang, Josephine H. Schamp, Brigitte C. Vanle Aldehyde dehydrogenase inhibition generates a reactive dopamine

metabolite autotoxic to dopamine neurons Parkinsonism & Related Disorders
https://doi.org/10.1016/S1353-8020(13)70019-1

[7] Philipp M. Amann, Katharina Czaja, Alexandr V. Bazhin, Ralph Rühl, Stefan
B. Eichmüller, Hans F. Merk, Jens M. Baron; LRAT Overexpression Diminishes
Intracellular Levels of Biologically Active Retinoids and Reduces Retinoid
Antitumor Efficacy in the Murine Melanoma B16F10 Cell Line. Skin Pharmacol
Physiol 1 June 2015; 28 (4): 205–212. https://doi.org/10.1159/000368806

[8] Chapter Three - Retinoid metabolism and functions mediated by retinoid
binding-proteins Joseph L. Napoli, Hong Sik Yoo Methods in Enzymology
https://doi.org/10.1016/bs.mie.2020.02.004

[9] Retinoic acid receptors and GATA transcription factors activate the
transcription of the human lecithin:retinol acyltransferase gene
Kun Cai [1], Lorraine J. Gudas The International Journal of Biochemistry & Cell
Biology https://doi.org/10.1016/j.biocel.2008.06.007

[10] Retinol and retinyl esters: biochemistry and physiology O'Byrne, Sheila M. et
al. Journal of Lipid Research, Volume 54, Issue 7, 1731 – 1743

[11] Kristoffer Ström, Thomas E. Gundersen, Ola Hansson, Stéphanie
Lucas, Céline Fernandez, Rune Blomhoff, Cecilia Holm Hormone-sensitive lipase
(HSL) is also a retinyl ester hydrolase: evidence from mice lacking HSL
https://doi.org/10.1096/fj.08-120923

[12] Mariel E. Toledo-Guzmán, Miguel Ibañez Hernández, Ángel A. Gómez-
Gallegos and Elizabeth Ortiz-Sánchez ALDH as a Stem Cell Marker in Solid
Tumors DOI: 10.2174/1574888X13666180810120012

[13][17] Radosław Januchowski [a], Karolina Wojtowicz [a], Maciej Zabel The role of
aldehyde dehydrogenase (ALDH) in cancer drug resistance Biomedicine &
Pharmacotherapy https://doi.org/10.1016/j.biopha.2013.04.005

[14] Ying, M., Wang, S., Sang, Y. et al. Regulation of glioblastoma stem cells by
retinoic acid: role for Notch pathway inhibition. Oncogene 30, 3454–3467 (2011).
https://doi.org/10.1038/onc.2011.58

[15] Monica Cojoc, Claudia Peitzsch, Ina Kurth, Franziska Trautmann, Leoni A.
Kunz-Schughart, Gennady D. Telegeev, Eduard A. Stakhovsky, John R.
Walker, Karl Simin, Stephen Lyle, Susanne Fuessel, Kati Erdmann, Manfred P.
Wirth, Mechthild Krause, Michael Baumann, Anna Dubrovska; Aldehyde
Dehydrogenase Is Regulated by β-catenin/TCF and Promotes Radioresistance in
Prostate Cancer Progenitor Cells. Cancer Res 1 April 2015; 75 (7): 1482–
1494. https://doi.org/10.1158/0008-5472.CAN-14-1924

[16] Young Chang Lim [a], Hyun Jung Kang [a], Young Sook Kim [a], Eun Chang Choi All-trans-retinoic acid inhibits growth of head and neck cancer stem cells by suppression of Wnt/β-catenin pathway European Journal of Cancer https://doi.org/10.1016/j.ejca.2012.04.013

[17] Jan S. Moreb, Amir Gabr, Govind R. Vartikar, Santosh Gowda, James R. Zucali and Dagmara Mohuczy Journal of Pharmacology and Experimental Therapeutics January 2005, 312 (1) 339-345; DOI: https://doi.org/10.1124/jpet.104.072496

[18] Duester, G. (2000), Families of retinoid dehydrogenases regulating vitamin A function. European Journal of Biochemistry, 267: 4315-4324. https://doi.org/10.1046/j.1432-1327.2000.01497.x

[19]
Teresa Karlsson [a], Anders Vahlquist [a], Natalia Kedishvili [b], Hans Törmä Biochemical and Biophysical Research Communications Volume 303, Issue 1, 28 March 2003, Pages 273-278 13-cis-Retinoic acid competitively inhibits 3α-hydroxysteroid oxidation by retinol dehydrogenase RoDH-4: a mechanism for its anti-androgenic effects in sebaceous glands?

[20] Stanczyk FZ. Diagnosis of hyperandrogenism: biochemical criteria. Best Pract Res Clin Endocrinol Metab. 2006 Jun;20(2):177-91. doi: 10.1016/j.beem.2006.03.007. PMID: 16772150.

[21] Nelson AM, Zhao W, Gilliland KL, Zaenglein AL, Liu W, Thiboutot DM. Temporal changes in gene expression in the skin of patients treated with isotretinoin provide insight into its mechanism of action. Dermatoendocrinol. 2009 May;1(3):177-87. doi: 10.4161/derm.1.3.8258. PMID: 20436886; PMCID: PMC2835911.

[22] Elaine M. Hull, Juan M. Dominguez Sexual behavior in male rodents Hormones and Behavior

Volume 52, Issue 1, June 2007, Pages 45-55 https://doi.org/10.1016/j.yhbeh.2007.03.030

[23] Cherrier, M.M., Craft, S. and Matsumoto, A.H. (2003), Cognitive Changes Associated With Supplementation of Testosterone or Dihydrotestosterone in Mildly Hypogonadal Men: A Preliminary Report. Journal of Andrology, 24: 568-576. https://doi.org/10.1002/j.1939-4640.2003.tb02708.x

Chapter 4 references

[1] Dr. B. D. Abbott, M. W. Harris, L. S. Birnbaum Etiology of retinoic acid-induced cleft palate varies with the embryonic
stage https://doi.org/10.1002/tera.1420400602

[2] Abdallah Abukhalil, Mai Yousef, Marwa Ammar, Weam Jaghama, Ni'meh Al-Shami, Hani Naseef, Abdullah Rabba, Practices, Efficacy, and Reported Side Effects Associated with Isotretinoin Treatment in Palestine, Patient Preference and Adherence, Volume 18, (487-501), (2024). https://doi.org/10.2147/PPA.S442436

[3] Marsha M. Dopheide [a], Russell E. Morgan Isotretinoin (13-cis-retinoic acid) alters learning and memory, but not anxiety-like behavior, in the adult rat https://doi.org/10.1016/j.pbb.2008.08.009

[4][8] Crandall J, Sakai Y, Zhang J, Koul O, Mineur Y, Crusio WE, McCaffery P. 13-cis-retinoic acid suppresses hippocampal cell division and hippocampal-dependent learning in mice. Proc Natl Acad Sci U S A. 2004 Apr 6;101(14):5111-6. doi: 10.1073/pnas.0306336101. Epub 2004 Mar 29. PMID: 15051884; PMCID: PMC387382.

[5] Marta U. Wołoszynowska-Fraser1, Azita Kouchmeshky2, and Peter McCaffery2 Vitamin A and Retinoic Acid in Cognition and Cognitive Disease https://doi.org/10.1146/annurev-nutr-122319-034227

[6] Afaf El-Ansary, Hanan A. Alfawaz, Abir Ben Bacha, Laila AL-Ayadhi, Assessing the COX-2/PGE2 Ratio and Anti-Nucleosome Autoantibodies as Biomarkers of Autism Spectrum Disorders: Using Combined ROC Curves to Improve Diagnostic Values, Current Issues in Molecular Biology, 46, 8, (8699-8709), (2024). https://doi.org/10.3390/cimb46080513

[7] Chenn A, Walsh CA. Regulation of cerebral cortical size by control of cell cycle exit in neural precursors. Science. 2002 Jul 19;297(5580):365-9. doi: 10.1126/science.1074192. PMID: 12130776.

[9] Alvaro Barrera-Ocampo, Johanna Gutierrez-Vargas, Luis Miguel Garcia-Segura, Gloria Patricia Cardona-Gómez Glycogen synthase kinase-3β/β-catenin signaling in the rat hypothalamus during the estrous cycle https://doi.org/10.1002/jnr.22816

[10] Tsukada M, Schröder M, Roos TC, Chandraratna RA, Reichert U, Merk HF, Orfanos CE, Zouboulis CC. 13-cis retinoic acid exerts its specific activity on human sebocytes through selective intracellular isomerization to all-trans retinoic acid and binding to retinoid acid receptors. J Invest Dermatol. 2000 Aug;115(2):321-7. doi: 10.1046/j.1523-1747.2000.00066.x. PMID: 10951254.

[11] Kimberly A. Maguschak and Kerry J. Ressler β-catenin is Required for Memory Consolidation Published online 2008 Sep 28. doi: 10.1038/nn.2198

[12] Szklarska D, Rzymski P. Is Lithium a Micronutrient? From Biological Activity and Epidemiological Observation to Food Fortification. Biol Trace Elem Res. 2019 May;189(1):18-27. doi: 10.1007/s12011-018-1455-2. Epub 2018 Jul 31. PMID: 30066063; PMCID: PMC6443601.

[13] Gin S. Malhi, Michelle Tanious, Pritha Das, Carissa M. Coulston & Michael Berk Potential Mechanisms of Action of Lithium in Bipolar Disorder Volume 27, pages 135–153, (2013)

[14] Wingo AP, Wingo TS, Harvey PD, Baldessarini RJ. Effects of lithium on cognitive performance: a meta-analysis. J Clin Psychiatry. 2009 Nov;70(11):1588-97. doi: 10.4088/JCP.08r04972. Epub 2009 Aug 11. PMID: 19689922.

[15] Xia MY, Zhao XY, Huang QL, Sun HY, Sun C, Yuan J, He C, Sun Y, Huang X, Kong W, Kong WJ. Activation of Wnt/β-catenin signaling by lithium chloride attenuates d-galactose-induced neurodegeneration in the auditory cortex of a rat model of aging. FEBS Open Bio. 2017 Apr 25;7(6):759-776. doi: 10.1002/2211-5463.12220. PMID: 28593132; PMCID: PMC5458451.

[16] Palmos, A.B., Duarte, R.R.R., Smeeth, D.M. et al. Lithium treatment and human hippocampal neurogenesis. Transl Psychiatry 11, 555 (2021). https://doi.org/10.1038/s41398-021-01695-y

[17] Young W. Review of Lithium Effects on Brain and Blood. Cell Transplantation. 2009;18(9):951-975. doi:10.3727/096368909X471251

[18] Gilbert C. The eye signs of vitamin A deficiency. Community Eye Health. 2013;26(84):66-7. PMID: 24782581; PMCID: PMC3936686.

[19] H. Maclean, M. Wright, D. Choi, M.J. Tidman, Abnormal night vision with isotretinoin therapy for acne, Clinical and Experimental Dermatology, Volume 20, Issue 1, 1 January 1995, Page 86, https://doi.org/10.1111/j.1365-2230.1995.tb01297.x

[20] Gamble MV, Mata NL, Tsin AT, Mertz JR, Blaner WS. Substrate specificities and 13-cis-retinoic acid inhibition of human, mouse and bovine cis-retinol dehydrogenases. Biochim Biophys Acta. 2000 Jan 3;1476(1):3-8. doi: 10.1016/s0167-4838(99)00232-0. PMID: 10606761.

[21] Chunfeng Lu, Songhua Li, Minghao Jin, Rapamycin Inhibits Light-Induced Necrosome Activation Occurring in Wild-Type, but not RPE65-Null, Mouse Retina, Investigative Opthalmology & Visual Science, 63, 13, (19), (2022). https://doi.org/10.1167/iovs.63.13.19

[22] Fraunfelder FW. Ocular side effects associated with isotretinoin. Drugs Today (Barc). 2004 Jan;40(1):23-7. doi: 10.1358/dot.2004.40.1.799435. PMID: 14988767.

[23] Botond Szabo Antiandrogenic effect of isotretinoin: Is the retina involved in mechanism of action? https://doi.org/10.1016/j.mehy.2007.03.026

[24] Ashton, A.; Clark, J.; Fedo, J.; Sementilli, A.; Fragoso, Y.D.; McCaffery, P. Retinoic Acid Signalling in the Pineal Gland Is Conserved across Mammalian Species and Its Transcriptional Activity Is Inhibited by Melatonin. Cells 2023, 12, 286. https://doi.org/10.3390/cells12020286

[25] Ashton, A., Stoney, P.N., Ransom, J. et al. Rhythmic Diurnal Synthesis and Signaling of Retinoic Acid in the Rat Pineal Gland and Its Action to Rapidly Downregulate ERK Phosphorylation. Mol Neurobiol 55, 8219–8235 (2018). https://doi.org/10.1007/s12035-018-0964-5

[26] Gisela Helfer, Alexander W. Ross, Laura Russell, Lynn M. Thomson, Kirsty D. Shearer, Timothy H. Goodman, Peter J. McCaffery, Peter J. Morgan, Photoperiod Regulates Vitamin A and Wnt/β-catenin Signaling in F344 Rats, Endocrinology, Volume 153, Issue 2, 1 February 2012, Pages 815–824, https://doi.org/10.1210/en.2011-1792

[27] Jennifer
N. Griffin, Daniel Pinali, Kaylan Olds, Na Lu, Lindsay Appleby, Louis Doan, Michelle A. Lane 13-Cis-retinoic acid decreases hypothalamic cell number in vitro https://doi.org/10.1016/j.neures.2010.08.003

[28] Masaru Katoh Regulation of WNT signaling molecules by retinoic acid during neuronal differentiation in NT2 cells: Threshold model of WNT action (Review) https://doi.org/10.3892/ijmm.10.6.683

[29] Batailler, M., Chesneau, D., Derouet, L. et al. Pineal-dependent increase of hypothalamic neurogenesis contributes to the timing of seasonal reproduction in sheep. Sci Rep 8, 6188 (2018). https://doi.org/10.1038/s41598-018-24381-4

[30]
C. Tocharus [a], Y. Puriboriboon [a], T. Junmanee [a], J. Tocharus [b], K. Ekthuwaprane [c], P. Govitrapong, Melatonin enhances adult rat hippocampal progenitor cell proliferation via ERK signaling pathway through melatonin receptor, https://doi.org/10.1016/j.neuroscience.2014.06.02

[31] James Crandall, Yasuo Sakai, Jinghua Zhang, +3, and Peter McCaffery Authors Info & Affiliations 13-cis-retinoic acid suppresses hippocampal cell division and hippocampal-dependent learning in mice https://doi.org/10.1073/pnas.0306336101

[32] Baris Sancak1 , Zeynep Ozdemir2 , Ozan Ozcan3 , Erkan Acar4 Melatonin Related Acneiform Lesions: A Case Report and Potential Mechanism, DOI:10.5152/pcp.2021.21234

[33] Sowon Bae1, Yoo Gyeong Yoon1,2, Ji Yea Kim3, In-Chul Park3, Sungkwan An1, Jae Ho Lee1, Seunghee Bae1 Melatonin increases growth properties in human dermal papilla spheroids by activating AKT/GSK3β/β-catenin signaling pathway PubMed 35607451

[34]
Yuliya Lytvyn PhD [a], Katherine McDonald MD [b], Asfandyar Mufti MD [b], Jennifer B eecker MD, CCFP (EM), FRCPC, FAAD Comparing the frequency of isotretinoin-induced hair loss at <0.5-mg/kg/d versus ≥0.5-mg/kg/d dosing in acne patients: A systematic review https://doi.org/10.1016/j.jdin.2022.01.002

[35] Thomas F. Ogle and Julian I. Kitay In Vitro Effects of Melatonin and Serotonin on Adrenal Steroidogenesis https://doi.org/10.3181/00379727-157-40000

[36] Mónica B. Frungieri, Artur Mayerhofer, Karina Zitta, Omar P. Pignataro, Ricardo S. Calandra, Silvia I. Gonzalez-Calvar, Direct Effect of Melatonin on Syrian Hamster Testes: Melatonin Subtype 1a Receptors, Inhibition of Androgen Production, and Interaction with the Local Corticotropin-Releasing Hormone System, Endocrinology, Volume 146, Issue 3, 1 March 2005, Pages 1541–1552, https://doi.org/10.1210/en.2004-0990

[37] Slavin J. Fiber and prebiotics: mechanisms and health benefits. Nutrients. 2013 Apr 22;5(4):1417-35. doi: 10.3390/nu5041417. PMID: 23609775; PMCID: PMC3705355.

[38] Crockett SD, Porter CQ, Martin CF, Sandler RS, Kappelman MD. Isotretinoin use and the risk of inflammatory bowel disease: a case-control study. Am J Gastroenterol. 2010 Sep;105(9):1986-93. doi: 10.1038/ajg.2010.124. Epub 2010 Mar 30. PMID: 20354506; PMCID: PMC3073620.

[39] Reddy, Deepa M.D.[1]; Siegel, Corey A. M.D.[2]; Sands, Bruce E. M.D., M.S.[2]; Kane, Sunanda M.D., M.S.P.H American Journal of Gastroenterology 101(7):p 1569-1573, July 2006. Possible Association Between Isotretinoin and Inflammatory Bowel Disease

[40] Bernstein CN, Nugent Z, Longobardi T, Blanchard JF. Isotretinoin is not associated with inflammatory bowel disease: a population-based case-control study. Am J Gastroenterol. 2009 Nov;104(11):2774-8. doi: 10.1038/ajg.2009.417. Epub 2009 Jul 21. PMID: 19623167.

[41] Tea Fevr,Sylvie Robine,Daniel Louvard &Joerg Huelsken Wnt/β-Catenin Is Essential for Intestinal Homeostasis and Maintenance of Intestinal Stem Cells https://doi.org/10.1128/MCB.01034-07

[42] Ordo´ n˜ ez-Mora´ n et al., 2015, Cancer Cell 28, 815–829 December 14, 2015 ª2015 Elsevier Inc. http://dx.doi.org/10.1016/j.ccell.2015.11.001

[43] Reniers DE, Howard JM. Isotretinoin-induced inflammatory bowel disease in an adolescent. Ann Pharmacother. 2001 Oct;35(10):1214-6. doi: 10.1345/aph.10368. PMID: 11675849.

[44] The Intestinal Crypt, A Prototype Stem Cell Compartment Clevers, Hans Cell, Volume 154, Issue 2, 274 - 284

[45] Daniel Pinto, Alex Gregorieff, Harry Begthel, and Hans Clevers Canonical Wnt signals are essential for homeostasis of the intestinal epithelium doi:10.1101/gad.267103

[46] Michael Bordonaro [1], Darina L. Lazarova [1], Alan C. Sartorelli The activation of beta-catenin by Wnt signaling mediates the effects of histone deacetylase inhibitors Experimental Cell Research Volume 313, Issue 8, 1 May 2007, Pages 1652-1666 https://doi.org/10.1016/j.yexcr.2007.02.008

 [47] Ware CB, Wang L, Mecham BH, Shen L, Nelson AM, Bar M, Lamba DA, Dauphin DS, Buckingham B, Askari B, Lim R, Tewari M, Gartler SM, Issa JP, Pavlidis P, Duan Z, Blau CA. Histone deacetylase inhibition elicits an evolutionarily conserved self-renewal program in embryonic stem cells. Cell Stem Cell. 2009 Apr 3;4(4):359-69. doi: 10.1016/j.stem.2009.03.001. PMID: 19341625; PMCID: PMC2719860.

[48] Gaoyang Liang · Olena Taranova · Kai Xia · Yi Zhang Butyrate Promotes Induced Pluripotent Stem Cell Generation Developmental BiologyVolume 285, Issue 33p25516-25521 August 2010

[49] Roy Hajjar,Carole S. Richard, andManuela M. Santos The role of butyrate in surgical and oncological outcomes in colorectal cancer https://doi.org/10.1152/ajpgi.00316.2020

Chapter 5 references

[1] Chunfeng Lu, Songhua Li, Minghao Jin, Rapamycin Inhibits Light-Induced Necrosome Activation Occurring in Wild-Type, but not RPE65-Null, Mouse Retina, Investigative Opthalmology & Visual Science, 63, 13, (19), (2022). https://doi.org/10.1167/iovs.63.13.19

[2] Fraunfelder FW. Ocular side effects associated with isotretinoin. Drugs Today (Barc). 2004 Jan;40(1):23-7. doi: 10.1358/dot.2004.40.1.799435. PMID: 14988767.

[3] Pavăl D, Rad F, Rusu R, Niculae AŞ, Colosi HA, Dobrescu I, Dronca E. Low Retinal Dehydrogenase 1 (RALDH1) Level in Prepubertal Boys with Autism Spectrum Disorder: A Possible Link to Dopamine Dysfunction? Clin Psychopharmacol Neurosci. 2017 Aug 31;15(3):229-236. doi: 10.9758/cpn.2017.15.3.229. PMID: 28783931; PMCID: PMC5565080.

[4] Modarai SR, Gupta A, Opdenaker LM, Kowash R, Masters G, Viswanathan V, Zhang T, Fields JZ, Boman BM. The anti-cancer effect of retinoic acid signaling in CRC occurs via decreased growth of ALDH+ colon cancer stem cells and increased differentiation of stem cells. Oncotarget. 2018 Oct 5;9(78):34658-34669. doi: 10.18632/oncotarget.26157. PMID: 30410666; PMCID: PMC6205182.

[5] Yu, RL., Tan, CH., Lu, YC. et al. Aldehyde dehydrogenase 2 is associated with cognitive functions in patients with Parkinson's disease. Sci Rep 6, 30424 (2016). https://doi.org/10.1038/srep30424

[6] Jonathan A. Doorn, Virginia R. Florang, Josephine H. Schamp, Brigitte C. Vanle Aldehyde dehydrogenase inhibition generates a reactive dopamine metabolite autotoxic to dopamine neurons https://doi.org/10.1016/S1353-8020(13)70019-1

[7][8] Seungju KimEun Young JangSang-Hoon SongJi Sun KimIn Soo RyuChul-Ho Jeong*Sooyeun Lee* Brain Microdialysis Coupled to LC-MS/MS Revealed That CVT-10216, a Selective Inhibitor of Aldehyde Dehydrogenase 2, Alters the Neurochemical and Behavioral Effects of Methamphetamine https://doi.org/10.1021/acschemneuro.1c00039

[9] C.P. Ford The role of D2-autoreceptors in regulating dopamine neuron activity and transmission https://doi.org/10.1016/j.neuroscience.2014.01.025

[10] Bello EP, Mateo Y, Gelman DM, Noaín D, Shin JH, Low MJ, Alvarez VA, Lovinger DM, Rubinstein M. Cocaine supersensitivity and enhanced motivation for reward in mice lacking dopamine D2 autoreceptors. Nat Neurosci. 2011 Jul 10;14(8):1033-8. doi: 10.1038/nn.2862. PMID: 21743470; PMCID: PMC3175737.

[11] Zald DH, Cowan RL, Riccardi P, Baldwin RM, Ansari MS, Li R, Shelby ES, Smith CE, McHugo M, Kessler RM. Midbrain dopamine receptor availability is

inversely associated with novelty-seeking traits in humans. J Neurosci. 2008 Dec 31;28(53):14372-8. doi: 10.1523/JNEUROSCI.2423-08.2008. PMID: 19118170; PMCID: PMC2748420.

[12] Wernicke, C., Hellmann, J., Finckh, U. et al. Chronic ethanol exposure changes dopamine D2 receptor splicing during retinoic acid-induced differentiation of human SH-SY5Y cells. Pharmacol. Rep 62, 649–663 (2010). https://doi.org/10.1016/S1734-1140(10)70322-4

[13] Kesby, J., Eyles, D., McGrath, J. et al. Dopamine, psychosis and schizophrenia: the widening gap between basic and clinical neuroscience. Transl Psychiatry 8, 30 (2018). https://doi.org/10.1038/s41398-017-0071-9

[14] Bryan K. Yamamoto Michael G. Bankson Amphetamine Neurotoxicity: Cause and Consequence of Oxidative Stress
DOI: 10.1615/CritRevNeurobiol.v17.i2.30

[15] Berman, S., Kuczenski, R., McCracken, J. et al. Potential adverse effects of amphetamine treatment on brain and behavior: a review. Mol Psychiatry 14, 123–142 (2009). https://doi.org/10.1038/mp.2008.90

[16] Du Toit Loots [a], Lodewyk J Mienie [a], Jacobus J Bergh [b], Cornelis J Van der Schyf Acetyl-L-carnitine prevents total body hydroxyl free radical and uric acid production induced by 1-methyl-4-phenyl-1,2,3,6-tetrahydropyridine (MPTP) in the rat https://doi.org/10.1016/j.lfs.2004.03.007

[17] Ahlam Alhusaini [a], Wedad Sarawi [a], Dareen Mattar [b], Amjad Abo-Hamad [c], Renad Almogren [d], Sara Alhumaidan [c], Ebtesam Alsultan [e], Shaikha Al saif [f], Iman Hasan [a], Emad Hassanein [g], Ayman Mahmoud Acetyl-L-carnitine and/or liposomal co-enzyme Q10 prevent propionic acid-induced neurotoxicity by modulating oxidative tissue injury, inflammation, and ALDH1A1-RA-RARα signaling in rats https://doi.org/10.1016/j.biopha.2022.113360

[18] Singh, S., Mishra, A. & Shukla, S. ALCAR Exerts Neuroprotective and Pro-Neurogenic Effects by Inhibition of Glial Activation and Oxidative Stress via Activation of the Wnt/β-catenin Signaling in Parkinsonian Rats. Mol Neurobiol 53, 4286–4301 (2016). https://doi.org/10.1007/s12035-015-9361-5

[19] Hart AM, Wilson AD, Montovani C, Smith C, Johnson M, Terenghi G, Youle M. Acetyl-l-carnitine: a pathogenesis based treatment for HIV-associated antiretroviral toxic neuropathy. AIDS. 2004 Jul 23;18(11):1549-60. doi: 10.1097/01.aids.0000131354.14408.fb. PMID: 15238773.

[20] Pennisi, M.; Lanza, G.; Cantone, M.; D'Amico, E.; Fisicaro, F.; Puglisi, V.; Vinciguerra, L.; Bella, R.; Vicari, E.; Malaguarnera, G. Acetyl-L-Carnitine in Dementia and Other Cognitive Disorders: A Critical Update. Nutrients 2020, 12, 1389. https://doi.org/10.3390/nu12051389

[21] Lisa Rebecca Otto, Vera Clemens, Berk Üsekes, Nicoleta Carmen Cosma, Francesca Regen, Julian Hellmann-Regen, Retinoid homeostasis in major depressive disorder, Translational Psychiatry, 13, 1, (2023). https://doi.org/10.1038/s41398-023-02362-0

Chapter 6 references

[1] Boldrini M, Underwood MD, Mann JJ, Arango V. Serotonin-1A autoreceptor binding in the dorsal raphe nucleus of depressed suicides. J Psychiatr Res. 2008 May;42(6):433-42. doi: 10.1016/j.jpsychires.2007.05.004. Epub 2007 Jun 15. PMID: 17574270; PMCID: PMC2268626.

[2] Alvaro L. Garcia-Garcia, Qingyuan Meng, Sarah Canetta, ..., Christoph Kellendonk, Alex Dranovsky, E. David Leonardo Serotonin Signaling through Prefrontal Cortex 5-HT1A Receptors during Adolescence Can Determine Baseline Mood-Related Behaviors http://dx.doi.org/10.1016/j.celrep.2017.01.021

[3] Lynne E. Rueter, Claude De Montigny, Pierre Blier In vivo electrophysiological assessment of the agonistic properties of flibanserin at pre- and postsynaptic 5-HT$_{1A}$ receptors in the rat brain https://doi.org/10.1002/(SICI)1098-2396(199808)29:4<392::AID-SYN11>3.0.CO;2-T

[4] O'Reilly KC, Trent S, Bailey SJ, Lane MA. 13-cis-Retinoic acid alters intracellular serotonin, increases 5-HT1A receptor, and serotonin reuptake transporter levels in vitro. Exp Biol Med (Maywood). 2007 Oct;232(9):1195-203. doi: 10.3181/0703-RM-83. PMID: 17895527.

[5] Emerson F. Harkin,Georges Nasrallah,Brice Le François andPaul R. Albert Transcriptional Regulation of the Human 5-HT1A Receptor Gene by Lithium: Role of Deaf1 and GSK3β https://doi.org/10.3390/ijms242115620

Chapter 7 references

[1][6] J. Douglas Bremner, M.D., Negar Fani, M.S., Ali Ashraf, M.D., John R. Votaw, Ph.D., Marijn E. Brummer, Ph.D., Thomas Cummins, M.D., Viola Vaccarino, M.D., Ph.D., Mark M. Goodman, Ph.D., Lai Reed, M.B.A., Sajid Siddiq, M.D., and Charles B. Nemeroff, M.D., Functional Brain Imaging

Alterations in Acne Patients Treated With Isotretinoin
https://doi.org/10.1176/appi.ajp.162.5.983

[2] Golec, K., Draps, M., Stark, R., Pluta, A., & Gola, M. (2021). Aberrant orbitofrontal cortex reactivity to erotic cues in Compulsive Sexual Behavior Disorder. Journal of Behavioral Addictions, 10(3), 646-656. https://doi.org/10.1556/2006.2021.00051

[3] Antoine Bechara, Antonio R. Damasio, Hanna Damasio, Steven W. Anderson Insensitivity to future consequences following damage to human prefrontal cortex https://doi.org/10.1016/0010-0277(94)90018-3

[4] Bremner JD, Vythilingam M, Vermetten E, Nazeer A, Adil J, Khan S, Staib LH, Charney DS. Reduced volume of orbitofrontal cortex in major depression. Biol Psychiatry. 2002 Feb 15;51(4):273-9. doi: 10.1016/s0006-3223(01)01336-1. PMID: 11958777.

[5] Elisabeth Wagner, Tuanlian Luo, Yasuo Sakai, Luis F. Parada, Ursula C. Dräger Retinoic acid delineates the topography of neuronal plasticity in postnatal cerebral cortex https://doi.org/10.1111/j.1460-9568.2006.04934.x

[7] The Thalamus Regulates Retinoic Acid Signaling and Development of Parvalbumin Interneurons in Postnatal Mouse Prefrontal Cortex Rachel Larsen, Alatheia Proue, Earl Parker Scott, Matthew Christiansen and Yasushi Nakagawa eNeuro 12 March 2019, 6 (1) ENEURO.0018-19.2019; https://doi.org/10.1523/ENEURO.0018-19.2019

[8] Alvaro L. Garcia-Garcia, Qingyuan Meng, Sarah Canetta, ..., Christoph Kellendonk, Alex Dranovsky, E. David Leonardo Serotonin Signaling through Prefrontal Cortex 5-HT1A Receptors during Adolescence Can Determine Baseline Mood-Related Behaviors http://dx.doi.org/10.1016/j.celrep.2017.01.021

[9] Brielle R. Ferguson Wen-Jun Gao*Wen-Jun Gao PV Interneurons: Critical Regulators of E/I Balance for Prefrontal Cortex-Dependent Behavior and Psychiatric Disorders https://doi.org/10.3389/fncir.2018.00037

[10] Urban, Kimberly R.,Layfield, Dylan M.,Griffin, Amy L. Transient inactivation of the medial prefrontal cortex impairs performance on a working memory-dependent conditional discrimination task. APA PsycNet Direct

[11] Nandakumar S. Narayanan· Mark Laubach Top-Down Control of Motor Cortex Ensembles by Dorsomedial Prefrontal Cortex Volume 52, Issue 5p921-931December 07, 2006

[12] D. Peleg-Raibstein, M.A. Pezze [1], B. Ferger [1], WN. Zhang, C.A. Murphy [1], J. Feldon, T. Bast Activation of dopaminergic neurotransmission in the medial prefrontal cortex

by N-methyl-d-aspartate stimulation of the ventral hippocampus in rats
https://doi.org/10.1016/j.neuroscience.2004.12.016

[13] Christina Chatzi,Thomas Brade,Gregg Duester Retinoic Acid Functions as a Key GABAergic Differentiation Signal in the Basal Ganglia
https://doi.org/10.1371/journal.pbio.1000609

[14] James E. Crandall, Timothy Goodman, Deirdre M. McCarthy, Gregg Duester, Pradeep G. Bhide, Ursula C. Dräger, Peter McCaffery Retinoic acid influences neuronal migration from the ganglionic eminence to the cerebral cortex https://doi.org/10.1111/j.1471-4159.2011.07471.x

[15] Huang C, Chen JT. Chronic retinoic acid treatment induces affective disorders by impairing the synaptic plasticity of the hippocampus. J Affect Disord. 2020 Sep 1;274:678-689. doi: 10.1016/j.jad.2020.05.114. Epub 2020 May 23. PMID: 32664002.

[16] Mami Takayama, Koichi Miyatake, Eisuke Nishida Identification and characterization of retinoic acid-responsive genes in mouse kidney development https://doi.org/10.1111/gtc.12163

[17] Lu, T., Pan, Y., Kao, SY. et al. Gene regulation and DNA damage in the ageing human brain. Nature 429, 883–891 (2004). https://doi.org/10.1038/nature02661

Chapter 8 references

[1] Markus Rieck, Wolfgang Meissner, Simone Ries, Sabine Müller-Brüsselbach and Rolf Müller Molecular Pharmacology November 2008, 74 (5) 1269-1277; DOI: https://doi.org/10.1124/mol.108.050625

[2] M.M. HALUZÍK1, 2, M. HALUZÍK PPAR-α and Insulin Sensitivity Physiol. Res. 55: 115-122, 2006

[3] C. Janani, B.D. Ranjitha Kumari PPAR gamma gene – A review https://doi.org/10.1016/j.dsx.2014.09.015

[4] Bart Staels, Jean Dallongeville, Johan Auwerx, Kristina Schoonjans, Eran Leitersdorf, and Jean-Charles Mechanism of Action of Fibrates on Lipid and Lipoprotein Metabolism https://doi.org/10.1161/01.CIR.98.19.2088

[5] Zech LA, Gross EG, Peck GL, Brewer HB. Changes in Plasma Cholesterol and Triglyceride Levels After Treatment With Oral Isotretinoin: A Prospective

Study. Arch Dermatol. 1983;119(12):987–993.
doi:10.1001/archderm.1983.01650360033009

[6] Tiangang Li, John Y. L. Chiang Regulation of Bile Acid and Cholesterol
Metabolism by PPARs https://doi.org/10.1155/2009/501739

[7] Nishit R. Trivedi [1][6], Zhaoyuan Cong [1][6], Amanda M. Nelson [1], Adam
J. Albert [2], Lorraine L. Rosamilia [3], Surendra Sivarajah [4], Kathryn
L. Gilliland [1], Wenlei Liu [5], David T. Mauger [5], Robert A. Gabbay [4], Diane
M. Thiboutot Peroxisome Proliferator-Activated Receptors Increase Human
Sebum Production https://doi.org/10.1038/sj.jid.5700336

[8] Gilles G. Lestringant md, Philippe M. Frossard phd, dsc, Mukesh Agarwal md,
Ibrahim H. Galadari md Variations in lipid and lipoprotein levels during
isotretinoin treatment for acne vulgaris with special emphasis on HDL-cholesterol
https://doi.org/10.1046/j.1365-4362.1997.00331.x

[9] Tsung-Yu Tsai, Han-Wen Liu, Yuan-Chen Chao, Yu-Chen Huang Effects of
isotretinoin on glucose metabolism in patients with acne: A systematic review
and meta-analysis https://doi.org/10.1111/ddg.14108

[10] Delphine Stoll [a], Christophe Binnert [a], Vincent Mooser [b], Luc Tappy Short-
term administration of isotretinoin elevates plasma triglyceride concentrations
without affecting insulin sensitivity in healthy humans
https://doi.org/10.1016/j.metabol.2003.07.006

[11] D. T. Ertugrul, A. S. Karadag, E. Tutal, K. O. Akin, Isotretinoin does not
induce insulin resistance in patients with acne, Clinical and Experimental
Dermatology, Volume 36, Issue 2, 1 March 2011, Pages 124–
128, https://doi.org/10.1111/j.1365-2230.2010.03915.x

[12] SOYUDURU, GONCA; ADIŞEN, ESRA ÖZSOY; ÖZER, İLKAY; and
AKSAKAL, AHMET BURHAN (2019) "The effect of isotretinoin on insulin
resistance and adipocytokine levels in acne vulgaris patients," Turkish Journal of
Medical Sciences: Vol. 49: No. 1, Article 35. https://doi.org/10.3906/sag-1806-44
Available at: https://journals.tubitak.gov.tr/medical/vol49/iss1/35

[13] Peng Zhang, Lei Tian, Jiayu Bao, Shang Li, Ao Li, Ya Wen, Jingyi
Wang, Ying Jie; Isotretinoin Impairs the Secretory Function of Meibomian Gland
Via the PPARγ Signaling Pathway. Invest. Ophthalmol. Vis.
Sci. 2022;63(3):29. https://doi.org/10.1167/iovs.63.3.29.

[14][30] SHORT TERM 13-cis-RETINOIC ACID TREATMENT AT
THERAPEUTIC DOSES ELEVATES EXPRESSION OF LEPTIN, GLUT4,
PPARγ AND aP2 IN RAT ADIPOSE TISSUE K. KRSKOVA-TYBITANCLOVA1,
D. MACEJOVA1, J. BRTKO1, M. BACULIKOVA1, O. KRIZANOVA2, S. ZORAD1
JOURNAL OF PHYSIOLOGY AND PHARMACOLOGY 2008, 59, 4, 731–743

[15] RDH10, RALDH2, and CRABP2 are required components of PPARγ-directed ATRA synthesis and signaling in human dendritic cells Gyöngyösi, Adrienn et al. Journal of Lipid Research, Volume 54, Issue 9, 2458 - 2474
[16][17] Madke B, Prasad K, Kar S. Isotretinoin-Induced Night Blindness. Indian J Dermatol. 2015 Jul-Aug;60(4):424. doi: 10.4103/0019-5154.160547. PMID: 26288455; PMCID: PMC4533586.

[18] Hempel, B., Crissman, M., Pari, S. et al. PPARα and PPARγ are expressed in midbrain dopamine neurons and modulate dopamine- and cannabinoid-mediated behavior in mice. Mol Psychiatry 28, 4203–4214 (2023).
https://doi.org/10.1038/s41380-023-02182-0

[19] Carroll, C.B., Zeissler, M.-.-L., Hanemann, C.O. and Zajicek, J.P. (2012), Δ9-tetrahydrocannabinol (Δ9-THC) exerts a direct neuroprotective effect in a human cell culture model of Parkinson's disease. Neuropathology and Applied Neurobiology, 38: 535-547. https://doi.org/10.1111/j.1365-2990.2011.01248.x

[20] Simona Scheggi [a,1], Miriam Melis [b,1], Marta De Felice [b], Sonia Aroni [b], Anna Lisa Muntoni [c], Teresa Pelliccia [a], Carla Gambarana [a], Maria Graziella De Montis [a,2], Marco Pistis PPARα modulation of mesolimbic dopamine transmission rescues depression-related behaviors
https://doi.org/10.1016/j.neuropharm.2016.07.024

[21] de Guglielmo, G., Melis, M., De Luca, M. et al. PPARγ Activation Attenuates Opioid Consumption and Modulates Mesolimbic Dopamine Transmission. Neuropsychopharmacol 40, 927–937 (2015).
https://doi.org/10.1038/npp.2014.268

[22] Lecarpentier, Yves, Claes, Victor, Vallée, Alexandre, Hébert, Jean-Louis, Interactions between PPAR Gamma and the Canonical Wnt/β-catenin Pathway in Type 2 Diabetes and Colon Cancer, PPAR Research, 2017, 5879090, 9 pages, 2017. https://doi.org/10.1155/2017/5879090

[23] Baykal Selçuk L, Aksu Arıca D, Baykal Şahin H, Yaylı S, Bahadır S. The prevalence of sacroiliitis in patients with acne vulgaris using isotretinoin. Cutan Ocul Toxicol. 2017 Jun;36(2):176-179. doi: 10.1080/15569527.2016.1237521. Epub 2016 Nov 16. PMID: 27764978.

[24] Namazi MR, Feily A. Hyperhomocysteinemia: Can't it account for retinoid-induced fracture proneness?. Indian J Dermatol Venereol Leprol 2010;76:186-187

[25] Takada, I., Kouzmenko, A. & Kato, S. Wnt and PPARγ signaling in osteoblastogenesis and adipogenesis. Nat Rev Rheumatol 5, 442–447 (2009).
https://doi.org/10.1038/nrrheum.2009.137

[26] Gustavo Duque, Wei Li, Christopher Vidal, Sandra Bermeo, Daniel Rivas, Janet Henderson, Pharmacological inhibition of PPARγ increases osteoblastogenesis and bone mass in male C57BL/6 mice, Journal of Bone and Mineral Research, Volume 28, Issue 3, 1 March 2013, Pages 639–648, https://doi.org/10.1002/jbmr.1782

[27] Lakota, K., Wei, J., Carns, M. et al. Levels of adiponectin, a marker for PPAR-gamma activity, correlate with skin fibrosis in systemic sclerosis: potential utility as biomarker? . Arthritis Res Ther 14, R102 (2012). https://doi.org/10.1186/ar3827

[28] Effects of isotretinoin on body mass index, serum adiponectin, leptin, and ghrelin levels in acne vulgaris patients Bengu Cevirgen Cemil,Havva Hilal Ayvaz,Gulfer Ozturk,Can Ergin,Havva Kaya Akıs,Muzeyyen Gonul,Ercan Arzuhal https://doi.org/10.5114/pdia.2016.56928

[29] Heliövaara MK, Remitz A, Reitamo S, Teppo AM, Karonen SL, Ebeling P. 13-cis-Retinoic acid therapy induces insulin resistance, regulates inflammatory parameters, and paradoxically increases serum adiponectin concentration. Metabolism. 2007 Jun;56(6):786-91. doi: 10.1016/j.metabol.2007.02.002. PMID: 17512311.

[31] Sedova, L., Seda, O., Krenova, D. et al. Isotretinoin and fenofibrate induce adiposity with distinct effect on metabolic profile in a rat model of the insulin resistance syndrome. Int J Obes 28, 719–725 (2004). https://doi.org/10.1038/sj.ijo.0802613

[32] Khalin E. Nisbett Graziano Pinna*Graziano Pinna Emerging Therapeutic Role of PPAR–α in Cognition and Emotions https://doi.org/10.3389/fphar.2018.00998

[33] Almeida, F.B.; Pinna, G.; Barros, H.M.T. The Role of HPA Axis and Allopregnanolone on the Neurobiology of Major Depressive Disorders and PTSD. Int. J. Mol. Sci. 2021, 22, 5495. https://doi.org/10.3390/ijms22115495

[34] G. Mattace Raso, E. Esposito, S. Vitiello, A. Iacono, A. Santoro, G. D'Agostino, O. Sasso, R. Russo, P. V. Piazza, A. Calignano, R. Meli Palmitoylethanolamide Stimulation Induces Allopregnanolone Synthesis in C6 Cells and Primary Astrocytes: Involvement of Peroxisome-Proliferator Activated Receptor-α https://doi.org/10.1111/j.1365-2826.2011.02152.x

[35] Sasso, Oscara; Russo, Robertoa; Vitiello, Sergiob,c; Raso, Giuseppina Mattacea; D'Agostino, Giuseppea; Iacono, Annaa; La Rana, Giovannaa; Vallée, Moniqueb,c; Cuzzocrea, Salvatored,e; Piazza, Pier Vincenzob,c; Meli, Rosariaa,*; Calignano, Antonio Implication of allopregnanolone in the

antinociceptive effect ofN-palmitoylethanolamide in acute or persistent pain DOI: 10.1016/j.pain.2011.08.010

[36][51] Graziano Pinna Role of PPAR-Allopregnanolone Signaling in Behavioral and Inflammatory Gut-Brain Axis Communications https://doi.org/10.1016/j.biopsych.2023.04.025

[37] Ann M. Rasmusson
Graziano Pinna [e], Prashni Paliwal [a c], David Weisman [b], Christopher Gottschalk [a b], Dennis Charney [f], John Krystal [a d], Alessandro Guidotti Allopregnanolone Levels in Women with Posttraumatic Stress Disorder https://doi.org/10.1016/j.biopsych.2006.03.026

[38] Ann M. Rasmusson, Matthew
W. King [a b c], Ivan Valovski [b d], Kristin Gregor [b c], Erica Scioli-Salter [a b c], Suzanne L. Pineles [a b c], Mohamed Hamouda [b d], Yael I. Nillni [a b c], George M. Anderson [e], Graziano Pinna Relationships between cerebrospinal fluid GABAergic neurosteroid levels and symptom severity in men with PTSD https://doi.org/10.1016/j.psyneuen.2018.11.027

[39] Teresa Karlsson [a], Anders Vahlquist [a], Natalia Kedishvili [b], Hans Törmä 13-cis-Retinoic acid competitively inhibits 3α-hydroxysteroid oxidation by retinol dehydrogenase RoDH-4: a mechanism for its anti-androgenic effects in sebaceous glands? https://doi.org/10.1016/S0006-291X(03)00332-2

[40] Nelson AM, Zhao W, Gilliland KL, Zaenglein AL, Liu W, Thiboutot DM. Temporal changes in gene expression in the skin of patients treated with isotretinoin provide insight into its mechanism of action. Dermatoendocrinol. 2009 May;1(3):177-87. doi: 10.4161/derm.1.3.8258. PMID: 20436886; PMCID: PMC2835911.

[41] E. Makrantonaki, C.C. Zouboulis, Testosterone metabolism to 5α-dihydrotestosterone and synthesis of sebaceous lipids is regulated by the peroxisome proliferator-activated receptor ligand linoleic acid in human sebocytes, British Journal of Dermatology, Volume 156, Issue 3, 1 March 2007, Pages 428–432, https://doi.org/10.1111/j.1365-2133.2006.07671.x

[42] Chen, MJ., Chou, CH., Chen, SU. et al. The effect of androgens on ovarian follicle maturation: Dihydrotestosterone suppress FSH-stimulated granulosa cell proliferation by upregulating PPARγ-dependent PTEN expression.. Sci Rep 5, 18319 (2016). https://doi.org/10.1038/srep18319

[43] R.L. Rosenfield, D. Deplewski, A. Kentsis, N. Ciletti; Mechanisms of Androgen Induction of Sebocyte Differentiation. Dermatology 1 July 1998; 196 (1): 43–46. https://doi.org/10.1159/000017864

[44] Inhibitory Effects of a Novel PPAR-γ Agonist MEKT1 on Pomc Expression/ACTH Secretion in AtT20 Cells Rehana Parvin, Erika Noro, Akiko Saito-Hakoda, Hiroki Shimada, Susumu Suzuki, Kyoko Shimizu, Hiroyuki Miyachi, Atsushi Yokoyama, Akira Sugawara https://doi.org/10.1155/2018/5346272

[45] Ayse Serap Karadag, Zennure Takci, Derun Taner Ertugrul, Serap Gunes Bilgili, Ragip Balahoroglu, Mumtaz Takir; The Effect of Different Doses of Isotretinoin on Pituitary Hormones. Dermatology 1 April 2015; 230 (4): 354–359. https://doi.org/10.1159/000375370

[46] Hunter Wessells [a], Dan Gralnek [b], Robert Dorr [c], Victor J Hruby [d], Mac E Hadley [e], Norman Levine Effect of an alpha-melanocyte stimulating hormone analog on penile erection and sexual desire in men with organic erectile dysfunction https://doi.org/10.1016/S0090-4295(00)00680-4

[47] Heaney, A., Fernando, M., Yong, W. et al. Functional PPAR-γ receptor is a novel therapeutic target for ACTH-secreting pituitary adenomas. Nat Med 8, 1281–1287 (2002). https://doi.org/10.1038/nm784

[48] Matrisciano, F.; Pinna, G. PPAR-α Hypermethylation in the Hippocampus of Mice Exposed to Social Isolation Stress Is Associated with Enhanced Neuroinflammation and Aggressive Behavior. Int. J. Mol. Sci. 2021, 22, 10678. https://doi.org/10.3390/ijms221910678

[49] Jiang X, Ye X, Guo W, Lu H, Gao Z. Inhibition of HDAC3 promotes ligand-independent PPARγ activation by protein acetylation. J Mol Endocrinol. 2014 Oct;53(2):191-200. doi: 10.1530/JME-14-0066. Epub 2014 Jun 30. PMID: 24982244; PMCID: PMC4391273.

[50] Roberto Russo [a], Carmen De Caro [a], Carmen Avagliano [a], Claudia Cristiano [a], Giovanna La Rana [a], Giuseppina Mattace Raso [a], Roberto Berni Canani [b], Rosaria Meli [a], Antonio Calignano Sodium butyrate and its synthetic amide derivative modulate nociceptive behaviors in mice https://doi.org/10.1016/j.phrs.2015.11.026

[52] Wang Zhang [a b], Ji-Hao Xu [a], Tao Yu [a], Qi-Kui Chen Effects of berberine and metformin on intestinal inflammation and gut microbiome composition in db/db mice https://doi.org/10.1016/j.biopha.2019.109131

Chapter 9 references

[1] Baxter NT, Schmidt AW, Venkataraman A, Kim KS, Waldron C, Schmidt TM. Dynamics of Human Gut Microbiota and Short-Chain Fatty Acids in Response to

Dietary Interventions with Three Fermentable Fibers. mBio. 2019 Jan 29;10(1):e02566-18. doi: 10.1128/mBio.02566-18. PMID: 30696735; PMCID: PMC6355990.

[2] Shin JH, Li RW, Gao Y, et al. Butyrate Induced IGF2 Activation Correlated with Distinct Chromatin Signatures Due to Histone Modification. Gene Regulation and Systems Biology. 2013;7. doi:10.4137/GRSB.S11243

[3] Bloemen, Johanne G. M.D.1,2; Schreinemacher, Marc H. M.D.1; de Bruine, Adriaan P. M.D., Ph.D.3; Buurman, Wim A. Ph.D.1; Bouvy, Nicole D. M.D., Ph.D.1; Dejong, Cornelis H. M.D., Ph.D.1. Butyrate Enemas Improve Intestinal Anastomotic Strength in a Rat Model. Diseases of the Colon & Rectum 53(7):p 1069-1075, July 2010. | DOI: 10.1007/DCR.0b013e3181d881b7

[4] Starches, Resistant Starches, the Gut Microflora and Human Health Anthony R Bird1, Ian L Brown2 and David L Topping1* 1CSIRO Health Sciences and Nutrition, GPO Box 10041, Kintore Avenue, Adelaide BC 5000, Australia 2Starch Australasia Ltd, 170, Epping Road Lane Cove 2066, Australia

[5] Baxter NT, Schmidt AW, Venkataraman A, Kim KS, Waldron C, Schmidt TM. Dynamics of Human Gut Microbiota and Short-Chain Fatty Acids in Response to Dietary Interventions with Three Fermentable Fibers. mBio. 2019 Jan 29;10(1):e02566-18. doi: 10.1128/mBio.02566-18. PMID: 30696735; PMCID: PMC6355990.

[6] Susan K. Raatz, Laura Idso, LuAnn K. Johnson, Matthew I. Jackson, Gerald F. Combs,Resistant starch analysis of commonly consumed potatoes: Content varies by cooking method and service temperature but not by variety,Food Chemistry,Volume 208,2016,Pages 297-300,ISSN 0308-8146,https://doi.org/10.1016/j.foodchem.2016.03.120.

[7] Effect of exercise and butyrate supplementation on microbiota composition and lipid metabolism in Journal of Endocrinology Chunxia Yu, Sujuan Liu, Liqin Chen, Jun Shen, Yanmei Niu, Tianyi Wang, Wanqi Zhang, and Li Fu DOI: https://doi.org/10.1530/JOE-19-0122

[8] Zhuang Li1,2, Chun-Xia Yi3, Saeed Katiraei4, Sander Kooijman1,2, Enchen Zhou1,2, Chih Kit Chung1, Yuanqing Gao3, José K van den Heuvel1,2, Onno C Meijer1,2, Jimmy F P Berbée1,2, Marieke Heijink5, Martin Giera5, Ko Willems van Dijk2,4, Albert K Groen6,7, Patrick C N Rensen1,2, Yanan Wang1,2,7 Butyrate reduces appetite and activates brown adipose tissue via the gut-brain neural circuit https://doi.org/10.1136/gutjnl-2017-314050

[9] Peng Zhang, Lei Tian, Jiayu Bao, Shang Li, Ao Li, Ya Wen, Jingyi Wang, Ying Jie; Isotretinoin Impairs the Secretory Function of Meibomian Gland Via the

PPARγ Signaling Pathway. Invest. Ophthalmol. Vis. Sci. 2022;63(3):29. https://doi.org/10.1167/iovs.63.3.29.

[10] Edenil Costa Aguilar, Josiane Fernandes da Silva, Juliana Maria Navia-Pelaez, Alda Jusceline Leonel, Lorrayne Gonçalves Lopes, Zélia Menezes-Garcia, Adaliene Versiani Matos Ferreira, Luciano dos Santos Aggum Capettini, Lilian G. Teixeira, Virginia Soares Lemos, Jacqueline I. Alvarez-Leite, Sodium butyrate modulates adipocyte expansion, adipogenesis, and insulin receptor signaling by upregulation of PPAR-γ in obese Apo E knockout mice,Nutrition,Volume 47,2018,Pages 75-82,ISSN 0899-9007,https://doi.org/10.1016/j.nut.2017.10.007.

[11] Ahlam Alhusaini, Wedad Sarawi, Dareen Mattar, Amjad Abo-Hamad, Renad Almogren, Sara Alhumaidan, Ebtesam Alsultan, Shaikha Alsaif, Iman Hasan, Emad Hassanein, Ayman Mahmoud, Acetyl-L-carnitine and/or liposomal co-enzyme Q10 prevent propionic acid-induced neurotoxicity by modulating oxidative tissue injury, inflammation, and ALDH1A1-RA-RARα signaling in rats, Biomedicine & Pharmacotherapy,Volume 153,2022,113360,ISSN 0753-3322,https://doi.org/10.1016/j.biopha.2022.113360.

[12] Ashton, A., Stoney, P.N., Ransom, J. et al. Rhythmic Diurnal Synthesis and Signaling of Retinoic Acid in the Rat Pineal Gland and Its Action to Rapidly Downregulate ERK Phosphorylation. Mol Neurobiol 55, 8219–8235 (2018). https://doi.org/10.1007/s12035-018-0964-5

[13] C. Tocharus, Y. Puriboriboon, T. Junmanee, J. Tocharus, K. Ekthuwapranee, P. Govitrapong, Melatonin enhances adult rat hippocampal progenitor cell proliferation via ERK signalling pathway through melatonin receptor, Neuroscience, Volume 275,2014,Pages 314-321,ISSN 0306-4522, https://doi.org/10.1016/j.neuroscience.2014.06.026.

[14] 13-cis-retinoic acid suppresses hippocampal cell division and hippocampal-dependent learning in miceJames Crandall, Yasuo Sakai, Jinghua Zhang, and Peter McCafferyAuthors Info & AffiliationsMarch 29, 2004101 (14) 5111-5116 https://doi.org/10.1073/pnas.0306336101

[15] Gisela Helfer, Alexander W. Ross, Laura Russell, Lynn M. Thomson, Kirsty D. Shearer, Timothy H. Goodman, Peter J. McCaffery, Peter J. Morgan, Photoperiod Regulates Vitamin A and Wnt/β-Catenin Signaling in F344 Rats, Endocrinology, Volume 153, Issue 2, 1 February 2012, Pages 815–824, https://doi.org/10.1210/en.2011-1792

[16] Gerardo Ramírez-Rodríguez, Nelly M. Vega-Rivera, Gloria Benítez-King, Mario Castro-García, Leonardo Ortíz-López,Melatonin supplementation delays the decline of adult hippocampal neurogenesis during normal aging of

mice,Neuroscience Letters,Volume 530, Issue 1,2012,Pages 53-58,ISSN 0304-3940,https://doi.org/10.1016/j.neulet.2012.09.045.

[17] Potes, Y.; Cachán-Vega, C.; Antuña, E.; García-González, C.; Menéndez-Coto, N.; Boga, J.A.; Gutiérrez-Rodríguez, J.; Bermúdez, M.; Sierra, V.; Vega-Naredo, I.; et al. Benefits of the Neurogenic Potential of Melatonin for Treating Neurological and Neuropsychiatric Disorders. Int. J. Mol. Sci. 2023, 24, 4803. https://doi.org/10.3390/ijms24054803

[18] Xia MY, Zhao XY, Huang QL, Sun HY, Sun C, Yuan J, He C, Sun Y, Huang X, Kong W, Kong WJ. Activation of Wnt/β-catenin signaling by lithium chloride attenuates d-galactose-induced neurodegeneration in the auditory cortex of a rat model of aging. FEBS Open Bio. 2017 Apr 25;7(6):759-776. doi: 10.1002/2211-5463.12220. PMID: 28593132; PMCID: PMC5458451.

[19] Palmos, A.B., Duarte, R.R.R., Smeeth, D.M. et al. Lithium treatment and human hippocampal neurogenesis. Transl Psychiatry 11, 555 (2021). https://doi.org/10.1038/s41398-021-01695-y

[20] Article Source: Chronic Microdose Lithium Treatment Prevented Memory Loss and Neurohistopathological Changes in a Transgenic Mouse Model of Alzheimer's Disease Nunes MA, Schöwe NM, Monteiro-Silva KC, Baraldi-Tornisielo T, Souza SIG, et al. (2015) Chronic Microdose Lithium Treatment Prevented Memory Loss and Neurohistopathological Changes in a Transgenic Mouse Model of Alzheimer's Disease. PLOS ONE 10(11): e0142267.https://doi.org/10.1371/journal.pone.0142267

[21] Palmos, A.B., Duarte, R.R.R., Smeeth, D.M. et al. Lithium treatment and human hippocampal neurogenesis. Transl Psychiatry 11, 555 (2021). https://doi.org/10.1038/s41398-021-01695-y

[22] https://www.nhs.uk/medicines/lithium/how-and-when-to-take-lithium/

[23] Bruce D. Lindsey, Kenneth Belitz, Charles A. Cravotta, Patricia L. Toccalino, Neil M. Dubrovsky,Lithium in groundwater used for drinking-water supply in the United States,Science of The Total Environment,Volume 767,2021,144691,ISSN 0048-9697,https://doi.org/10.1016/j.scitotenv.2020.144691.

[24] Gitlin, M. Lithium side effects and toxicity: prevalence and management strategies. Int J Bipolar Disord 4, 27 (2016). https://doi.org/10.1186/s40345-016-0068-y

[25] Arnold Orwin, Hair loss following lithium therapy, British Journal of Dermatology, Volume 108, Issue 4, 1 April 1983, Pages 503–504, https://doi.org/10.1111/j.1365-2133.1983.tb04607.x

[26] Yucel G, Van Arnam J, Means PC, Huntzicker E, Altindag B, Lara MF, Yuan J, Kuo C, Oro AE. Partial proteasome inhibitors induce hair follicle growth by stabilizing β-catenin. Stem Cells. 2014 Jan;32(1):85-92. doi: 10.1002/stem.1525. PMID: 23963711; PMCID: PMC4116182.

[27] Microdose Lithium Treatment Stabilized Cognitive Impairment in Patients with Alzheimer's Disease Andrade Nunes, Marielza; Araujo Viel, Tania; Sousa Buck, Hudson Bentham Science Publishers https://doi.org/10.2174/156720513804871354

[28] Yu, C., Liu, S., Chen, L., Shen, J., Niu, Y., Wang, T., Zhang, W., & Fu, L. (2019). Effect of exercise and butyrate supplementation on microbiota composition and lipid metabolism. Journal of Endocrinology, 243(2), 125-135. Retrieved Nov 9, 2024, from https://doi.org/10.1530/JOE-19-0122

[29] Low-dose lithium impact in an addiction treatment setting Sudhir Gadh Personalized Medicine in Psychiatry https://doi.org/10.1016/j.pmip.2020.100059

[30] Debidas Ghosh, Arnab Chaudhuri, Narendra M. Biswas, Pradip K. Ghosh, Effects of lithium chloride on testicular steroidogenic and gametogenic functions in mature male albino rats,Life Sciences,Volume 46, Issue 2,1990,Pages 127-137,ISSN 0024-3205,https://doi.org/10.1016/0024-3205(90)90045-S.

[31] Son P, Lewis L. Hyperhomocysteinemia. 2022 May 8. In: StatPearls [Internet]. Treasure Island (FL): StatPearls Publishing; 2024 Jan–. PMID: 32119295.

[32] Hyun Jung Kim PhD, Seung Min Lee MD, BS, Jong Suk Lee MD, PhD, Sung Yul Lee MD, PhD, Euy Hyun Chung MD, MS, Moon Kyun Cho MD, PhD, Sang Hoon Lee MD, PhD, Jung Eun Kim MD, PhD Homocysteine, folic acid, and vitamin B12 levels in patients on isotretinoin therapy for acne vulgaris: A meta-analysis https://doi.org/10.1111/jocd.13059

[33] J. Douglas Bremner,Isotretinoin and neuropsychiatric side effects: Continued vigilance is needed,Journal of Affective Disorders Reports,Volume 6,2021,100230,ISSN 2666-9153, https://doi.org/10.1016/j.jadr.2021.100230.

[34] Dezhi Kang et al. ,Vitamin B12 modulates the transcriptome of the skin microbiota in acne pathogenesis.Sci. Transl. Med.7,293ra103-293ra103(2015).DOI:10.1126/scitranslmed.aab2009

[35] Feily A. Successful Treatment of Isotretinoin Induced Musculoskeletal Pain by Vitamin B12 and Folic Acid. Open Access Maced J Med Sci. 2019 Oct 10;7(21):3726-3727. doi: 10.3889/oamjms.2019.799. PMID: 32010406; PMCID: PMC6986527.

[36] Janda, C., Dang, L., You, C. et al. Surrogate Wnt agonists that phenocopy canonical Wnt and β-catenin signalling. Nature **545**, 234–237 (2017). https://doi.org/10.1038/nature22306

[37] Walter Krugluger, Karl Stiefsohn, Katharina Laciak, Karl Moser, Claudia Moser Vitamin B12 Activates the Wnt-Pathway in Human Hair Follicle Cells by Induction of β-Catenin and Inhibition of Glycogensynthase Kinase-3 Transcription doi:10.4236/jcdsa.2011.12004 Published Online June 2011 (http://www.SciRP.org/journal/jcdsa)

[38] Ayman Abdelmaksoud, Aleksandra Vojvodic, Erhan Ayhan, Süleyman Dönmezdil, Tatjana Vlaskovic Jovicevic, Petar Vojvodic, Torello Lotti, Michelangelo Vestita Depression, isotretinoin, and folic acid: A practical review https://doi.org/10.1111/dth.13104

[39] Budni J, Lobato KR, Binfaré RW, et al. Involvement of PI3K, GSK-3β and PPARγ in the antidepressant-like effect of folic acid in the forced swimming test in mice. Journal of Psychopharmacology. 2012;26(5):714-723. doi:10.1177/0269881111424456

[40] A. Coppen, S. Chaudhry, C. Swade, Folic acid enhances lithium prophylaxis, Journal of Affective Disorders, Volume 10, Issue 1, 1986, Pages 9-13, ISSN 0165-0327, https://doi.org/10.1016/0165-0327(86)90043-1.

[41] Schrauzer, G.N., Shrestha, K.P. & Flores-Arce, M.F. Lithium in scalp hair of adults, students, and violent criminals. Biol Trace Elem Res **34**, 161–176 (1992). https://doi.org/10.1007/BF02785244

[42] Berridge MJ. Inositol Trisphosphate, Calcium, Lithium, and Cell Signaling. JAMA. 1989;262(13):1834–1841. doi:10.1001/jama.1989.03430130110043

[43] S.J.R. Allan, G.M. Kavanagh, R.M. Herd, J.A. Savin The effect of inositol supplements on the psoriasis of patients taking lithium: a

randomized, placebo-controlled trial https://doi.org/10.1111/j.1365-2133.2004.05822.x

[44] L. JANIRI1, F. D'AMBROSIO2, C. DI LORENZO Combined treatment of myo-inositol and d-chiro-inositol (80:1) as a therapeutic approach to restore inositol eumetabolism in patients with bipolar disorder taking lithium and valproic acid European Review for Medical and Pharmacological Sciences 2021; 25: 5483-5489

[46] W. Wallace Harrington, Christy S. Britt, Joan G. Wilson, Naphtali O. Milliken, Jane G. Binz, David C. Lobe, William R. Oliver, Michael C. Lewis, Diane M. Ignar The Effect of PPARα, PPARδ, PPARγ, and PPARpan Agonists on Body Weight, Body Mass, and Serum Lipid Profiles in Diet-Induced Obese AKR/J Mice https://doi.org/10.1155/2007/97125

[47] Nishit R. Trivedi [1,6], Zhaoyuan Cong [1,6], Amanda M. Nelson [1], Adam J. Albert [2], Lorraine L. Rosamilia [3], Surendra Sivarajah [4], Kathryn L. Gilliland [1], Wenlei Liu [5], David T. Mauger [5], Robert A. Gabbay [4], Diane M. Thiboutot Peroxisome Proliferator-Activated Receptors Increase Human Sebum Production https://doi.org/10.1038/sj.jid.5700336

[48] Peng Zhang, Lei Tian, Jiayu Bao, Shang Li, Ao Li, Ya Wen, Jingyi Wang, Ying Jie; Isotretinoin Impairs the Secretory Function of Meibomian Gland Via the PPARγ Signaling Pathway. Invest. Ophthalmol. Vis. Sci. 2022;63(3):29. https://doi.org/10.1167/iovs.63.3.29.

[49] Gupta, M., Mahajan, V.K., Mehta, K.S. et al. Peroxisome proliferator-activated receptors (PPARs) and PPAR agonists: the 'future' in dermatology therapeutics?. Arch Dermatol Res **307**, 767–780 (2015). https://doi.org/10.1007/s00403-015-1571-1

[50] Rosenfield RL, Deplewski D, Kentsis A, Ciletti N. Mechanisms of androgen induction of sebocyte differentiation. Dermatology. 1998;196(1):43-6. doi: 10.1159/000017864. PMID: 9557223.

[51] Imperato-McGinley J, Gautier T, Cai LQ, Yee B, Epstein J, Pochi P. The androgen control of sebum production. Studies of subjects with dihydrotestosterone deficiency and complete androgen insensitivity. J

Clin Endocrinol Metab. 1993 Feb;76(2):524-8. doi: 10.1210/jcem.76.2.8381804. PMID: 8381804.

[52]
Teresa Karlsson [a], Anders Vahlquist [a], Natalia Kedishvili [b], Hans Törmä 13-cis-Retinoic acid competitively inhibits 3α-hydroxysteroid oxidation by retinol dehydrogenase RoDH-4: a mechanism for its anti-androgenic effects in sebaceous glands? https://doi.org/10.1016/S0006-291X(03)00332-2

[53] Cermak JM, Krenzer KL, Sullivan RM, Dana MR, Sullivan DA. Is complete androgen insensitivity syndrome associated with alterations in the meibomian gland and ocular surface? Cornea. 2003 Aug;22(6):516-21. doi: 10.1097/00003226-200308000-00006. PMID: 12883343.

[54] Marwa A.A. Ibrahim, Walaa M. Elwan Role of topical dehydroepiandrosterone in ameliorating isotretinoin-induced Meibomian gland dysfunction in adult male albino rat https://doi.org/10.1016/j.aanat.2017.01.007

[55] Y.T. Konttinen [a b], V. Stegajev [a], A. Al-Samadi [a], P. Porola [a], J. Hietanen [c d], M. Ainola Sjögren's syndome and extragonadal sex steroid formation: A clue to a better disease control? https://doi.org/10.1016/j.jsbmb.2014.08.014

[56] Chen, F.L., Yang, Z.H., Liu, Y. et al. Berberine inhibits the expression of TNFα, MCP-1, and IL-6 in AcLDL-stimulated macrophages through PPARγ pathway. Endocr **33**, 331–337 (2008). https://doi.org/10.1007/s12020-008-9089-3

[57] Yan Yao, Jing Zuo, Li Chen, Yuegang Wei Combination of metformin and berberine represses the apoptosis of sebocytes in high-fat diet-induced diabetic hamsters and an insulin-treated human cell line https://doi.org/10.1002/cbf.3504

[58] Khalin E. NisbettGraziano Pinna*Graziano Pinna* Emerging Therapeutic Role of PPAR–α in Cognition and Emotions Front. Pharmacol., 02 October 2018 Sec. Neuropharmacology https://doi.org/10.3389/fphar.2018.00998

[59] Almeida, F.B.; Pinna, G.; Barros, H.M.T. The Role of HPA Axis and Allopregnanolone on the Neurobiology of Major Depressive Disorders and PTSD. Int. J. Mol. Sci. **2021**, 22, 5495. https://doi.org/10.3390/ijms22115495

[60] Rohini Pakhiddey a* , Shipra Paul b , Ashish K. Mandal c , Vijay Kumar Epidermal androgen receptors in acne vulgaris patients before and following oral isotretinoin http://dx.doi.org/10.1016/j.jasi.2015.04.002

[61] Boudou P, Soliman H, Chivot M, Villette JM, Vexiau P, Belanger A, Fiet J. Effect of oral isotretinoin treatment on skin androgen receptor levels in male acneic patients. J Clin Endocrinol Metab. 1995 Apr;80(4):1158-61. doi: 10.1210/jcem.80.4.7714084. PMID: 7714084.

[62] Song LN, Herrell R, Byers S, Shah S, Wilson EM, Gelmann EP. Beta-catenin binds to the activation function 2 region of the androgen receptor and modulates the effects of the N-terminal domain and TIF2 on ligand-dependent transcription. Mol Cell Biol. 2003 Mar;23(5):1674-87. doi: 10.1128/MCB.23.5.1674-1687.2003. PMID: 12588987; PMCID: PMC151689.

[63] Kraemer WJ, Spiering BA, Volek JS, Ratamess NA, Sharman MJ, Rubin MR, French DN, Silvestre R, Hatfield DL, Van Heest JL, Vingren JL, Judelson DA, Deschenes MR, Maresh CM. Androgenic responses to resistance exercise: effects of feeding and L-carnitine. Med Sci Sports Exerc. 2006 Jul;38(7):1288-96. doi: 10.1249/01.mss.0000227314.85728.35. Erratum in: Med Sci Sports Exerc. 2006 Oct;38(10):1861. PMID: 16826026.

[64] Bamman MM, Shipp JR, Jiang J, Gower BA, Hunter GR, Goodman A, McLafferty CL Jr, Urban RJ. Mechanical load increases muscle IGF-I and androgen receptor mRNA concentrations in humans. Am J Physiol Endocrinol Metab. 2001 Mar;280(3):E383-90. doi: 10.1152/ajpendo.2001.280.3.E383. PMID: 11171591.

[65] G. Cavallini a, S. Caracciolo b, G. Vitali a, F. Modenini a, G. Biagiotti Carnitine versus androgen administration in the treatment of sexual dysfunction, depressed mood, and fatigue associated with male aging https://doi.org/10.1016/j.urology.2003.11.009

[66] Pourshahidi, S., Shamshiri, A.R., Derakhshan, S. et al. The Effect of Acetyl-L-Carnitine (ALCAR) on Peripheral Nerve Regeneration in Animal Models: A Systematic Review. Neurochem Res **48**, 2335–2344 (2023). https://doi.org/10.1007/s11064-023-03911-1